Blood Type RH Negative Diet Book

Eating for Your Unique Blood Type: RH Negative Diet Strategies for Better Living

Taylor D. Rivers

INTRODUCTION

Welcome to The Blood Type RH Negative Diet, a comprehensive guide crafted specifically for individuals with RH negative blood types who seek to optimize their health and well-being through targeted nutrition. In recent years, dietary approaches tailored to individual blood types have gained popularity, and this book focuses on one such unique and often misunderstood group: those with RH negative blood.

Our blood type is more than just a marker for blood transfusions; it plays a pivotal role in our overall health and metabolism. Blood Type RH negative, a rare and intriguing classification, has distinct characteristics that may influence how our bodies respond to different foods and dietary patterns. While mainstream dietary advice often provides one-size-fits-all solutions, this book delves into the specific needs and benefits of the RH negative diet, offering a personalized approach to nutrition.

The Blood Type RH Negative Diet is grounded in the premise that our unique blood types affect how we metabolize foods and nutrients. The RH negative factor is believed to interact with various aspects of our digestive and immune systems, influencing our optimal dietary choices. By understanding these interactions, we can tailor our diet to enhance our health, boost our energy levels, and support overall well-being.

Individuals with RH negative blood types often experience unique challenges and opportunities in their nutritional journey. This book aims to address these specific needs by offering a curated selection of foods and recipes that align with the principles of the RH negative diet. Whether you are new to this approach or seeking to refine your current eating habits, this guide provides the tools and knowledge to help you succeed.

Embark on this journey with confidence, knowing that you are taking a proactive step towards a healthier, more balanced lifestyle. Let this book be your trusted companion as you explore the benefits of the Blood Type RH Negative Diet and discover how tailored nutrition can lead to a vibrant and fulfilling life.

TABLE OF CONTENTS

INTRODUCTION..2

1.1 Understanding Blood Type RH Negative..6

1.2 The Science Behind Blood Type Diets... 8

1.3 Why Focus on RH Negative?...11

Chapter 1: The RH Negative Diet Explained................................... **14**

2.1 The Role of Blood Type in Metabolism..14

2.2 Key Principles of the RH Negative Diet... 17

2.3 Benefits of Following the RH Negative Diet...................................... 18

Chapter 2: Foods to Embrace...**19**

3.1 Ideal Foods for RH Negative Blood Types...19

3.2 Nutritional Benefits of These Foods..20

Chapter 3: Foods to Avoid.. **21**

4.1 Foods That May Cause Issues for RH Negative Individuals................21

4.2 Understanding Food Sensitivities and Reactions...............................22

4.3 Alternatives and Substitutions...24

Chapter 4: Sample Meal Plans... **26**

5.1 7-Day Meal Plan for Beginners.. 26

5.2 Advanced Meal Planning for Long-Term Success.............................29

Chapter 5: Recipes for Every Meal.. **32**

6.1 Breakfast.. **32**

6.1.1 Berry and Spinach Smoothie...32

6.1.2 Quinoa Breakfast Bowl..33

6.1.3 Avocado and Egg Toast.. 35

6.1.4 Greek Yogurt with Nuts and Honey... 37

6.1.5 Sweet Potato Hash..39

6.1.6 Chia Pudding with Almond Milk... 41

6.1.7 Oatmeal with Apple and Cinnamon..43

6.1.8 Veggie Omelette...45

6.1.9 Smoothie Bowl with Toppings..47

6.1.10 Coconut Flour Pancakes...49

6.1.11 Egg and Veggie Breakfast Muffins..51

6.1.12 Buckwheat Porridge...53

6.1.13 Pumpkin Spice Smoothie..55

6.1.14 Almond Flour Waffles..56

6.1.15 Smoked Salmon and Avocado Wrap..58

6.2 Lunch..**60**

6.2.1 Quinoa and Black Bean Salad..60

6.2.2 Grilled Chicken and Veggie Wrap...63

6.2.3 Mediterranean Chickpea Salad..65

6.2.4 Sweet Potato and Kale Salad...67

6.2.5 Lentil Soup...69

6.2.6 Turkey and Avocado Lettuce Wraps..71

6.2.7 Stuffed Bell Peppers..73

6.2.8 Asian Noodle Salad..75

6.2.9 Cauliflower Rice Bowl...77

6.2.10 Chicken and Spinach Soup...79

6.2.11 Avocado and Chickpea Salad..81

6.2.12 Tuna Salad Stuffed Tomatoes...83

6.2.13 Zucchini Noodles with Pesto..85

6.2.14 Spicy Black Bean and Corn Salad..87

6.2.15 Butternut Squash and Lentil Curry...89

6.3 Dinner..**91**

6.3.1 Grilled Salmon with Asparagus...91

6.3.2 Chicken Stir-Fry..93

6.3.3 Beef and Broccoli...95

6.3.4 Stuffed Acorn Squash...97

6.3.5 Lemon Herb Chicken Thighs..99

6.3.6 Eggplant Parmesan...101

6.3.7 Shrimp and Vegetable Skewers.......................................104

6.3.8 Turkey Meatballs with Zucchini Noodles......................106

6.3.9 Baked Cod with Spinach and Tomatoes........................108

6.3.10 Spaghetti Squash with Marinara Sauce.......................110

6.3.11 Chili with Beans...112

6.3.12 Thai Coconut Curry..114

6.3.13 Roasted Vegetable Medley...116

6.3.14 Grilled Portobello Mushrooms with Garlic.................118

6.3.15 Lamb Chops with Mint Yogurt Sauce.........................120

6.4 Snacks...**122**

6.4.1 Hummus with Veggie Sticks...122

6.4.2 Apple Slices with Almond Butter..................................124

6.4.3 Greek Yogurt with Honey and Nuts..............................126

6.4.4 Homemade Trail Mix...128

6.4.5 Rice Cakes with Avocado...130

6.4.6 Cucumber and Cream Cheese Bites...............................132

6.4.7 Baked Sweet Potato Chips...134

6.4.8 Protein Balls...136

6.4.9 Edamame with Sea Salt...138

6.4.10 Stuffed Dates..140

6.4.11 Chia Seed Pudding..142

6.4.12 Celery Sticks with Peanut Butter.................................144

6.4.13 Homemade Popcorn..146

6.4.14 Fruit Smoothie..148

6.4.15 Spiced Nuts...150

6.5 Desserts..**152**

6.5.1 Berry Coconut Crumble...152

6.5.2 Almond Flour Brownies...154

6.5.3 Chocolate Chia Pudding...156

6.5.4 Baked Apples with Cinnamon...158

6.5.5 Avocado Chocolate Mousse..160

6.5.6 Frozen Banana Bites.. 161

6.5.7 Coconut Macaroons...163

6.5.8 Pumpkin Spice Muffins...165

6.5.9 Fruit Sorbet..167

6.5.10 Date and Nut Energy Balls.. 169

6.5.11 Greek Yogurt Parfait..171

6.5.12 Apple Cinnamon Oat Bars.. 172

6.5.13 Raspberry Lemon Bars...174

6.5.14 Chia and Fruit Salad..176

6.5.15 Dark Chocolate Almond Clusters..................................178

Chapter 6: Lifestyle and Wellness Tips....................................180

7.1 Incorporating Exercise for Optimal Health......................... 180

7.2 Stress Management Techniques..182

7.3 Sleep and Its Impact on Your Diet......................................185

Chapter 7: Troubleshooting and FAQs.....................................188

8.1 Common Challenges and Solutions.....................................189

8.2 How to Adjust the Diet for Specific Health Conditions......191

8.3 Final Though...193

1.1 Understanding Blood Type RH Negative

Blood type is a critical aspect of our physiology, influencing not only our compatibility for blood transfusions but also our overall health and nutritional needs. Among the various blood types, RH negative is relatively rare and holds unique characteristics that can impact how we interact with different foods and dietary patterns.

What is RH Negative Blood?

Blood type classification is determined by the presence or absence of specific antigens on the surface of red blood cells. The RH factor is one such antigen, which can be either present (RH positive) or absent (RH negative). If your blood lacks the RH antigen, you are classified as RH negative.

This absence of the RH antigen can influence several aspects of your health. For instance, individuals with RH negative blood may have a different immune response compared to those with RH positive blood. This variation can affect how the body processes certain foods, which is why understanding your blood type can be crucial for optimizing your diet.

Prevalence and Genetic Factors

RH negative blood is less common than RH positive blood, with varying prevalence across different populations and ethnic groups. In some populations, such as those of European descent, the frequency of RH negative individuals is higher, while in others, it is relatively rare. This genetic trait is inherited, meaning it is passed down through families, and understanding its implications can help in tailoring health and dietary recommendations.

Understanding your blood type, particularly if you are RH negative, provides valuable insights into how your body interacts with different foods and nutrients. This knowledge can empower you to make informed dietary choices that support your unique health needs. As you explore the Blood Type RH Negative Diet, keep in mind that this personalized approach is designed to help you achieve optimal health by aligning your diet with your blood type's specific characteristics.

By comprehending the nuances of RH negative blood and its implications, you are taking an important step towards a more tailored and effective approach to nutrition and health.

1.2 The Science Behind Blood Type Diets

The concept of blood type diets is based on the idea that our blood type influences how our bodies metabolize different foods and nutrients. This approach was popularized by Dr. Peter D'Adamo in his book Eat Right 4 Your Type, which proposes that specific diets tailored to individual blood types can lead to better health and well-being. The science behind these diets is multifaceted and involves several key principles.

Blood Type and Digestion

The core idea behind blood type diets is that each blood type has a unique set of antigens and proteins that interact with dietary components. These interactions can affect digestive efficiency and nutrient absorption. For example:

- **Lectins:** These are proteins found in various foods that can interact with blood type antigens. Some researchers suggest that certain lectins may agglutinate (clump together) with red blood cells, potentially leading to digestive issues or inflammation. The blood type diet recommends avoiding foods with lectins that may be incompatible with your blood type.

Metabolism and Food Sensitivities

Different blood types may exhibit varying responses to the same foods due to differences in metabolic processes and immune responses. For example:

- **Blood Type A:** Individuals with this blood type are thought to have a more sensitive immune system and may benefit from a diet rich in vegetables and lean proteins, while avoiding dairy and red meat.
- **Blood Type O:** This blood type is often associated with a more robust digestive system that can handle higher levels of protein and fats but may struggle with grains and legumes.

- **Blood Type B and AB:** These blood types are believed to have unique dietary needs, with Type B benefiting from a balanced diet that includes dairy and a variety of meats, while Type AB may require a more varied diet with both animal and plant-based foods.

Immunological Considerations

The science behind blood type diets also considers the role of blood type antigens in immune function. Each blood type has distinct antigens on the surface of red blood cells, which may interact with immune cells and affect how the body responds to various dietary components. The theory suggests that consuming foods that are compatible with your blood type can support immune health and reduce inflammation.

Research and Controversies

While the blood type diet has gained popularity, it is important to note that scientific support for these diets is mixed. Some studies have shown that people following blood type-specific diets experience health benefits, while others have found no significant differences compared to general dietary guidelines. The lack of large-scale, peer-reviewed studies makes it challenging to conclusively determine the effectiveness of blood type diets.

Integrating the Science

Despite the ongoing debate, many individuals find personalized approaches to nutrition beneficial. The blood type diet offers a framework for understanding how dietary choices might interact with one's genetic predispositions. For those interested in exploring this approach, it is advisable to consider it as part of a broader, evidence-based nutritional strategy that includes balanced eating, regular exercise, and overall health management.

The science behind blood type diets explores the interactions between blood type antigens, digestive processes, and immune function. While the concept offers intriguing insights into personalized nutrition, the scientific community continues to debate its efficacy. For those interested in the blood type diet, it provides a potential framework for tailoring dietary choices to individual needs, but it should be approached with an understanding of its current scientific standing and complemented with other health practices.

1.3 Why Focus on RH Negative?

Focusing on the RH negative blood type offers a unique perspective on personalized nutrition and health management. While blood type diets generally address dietary needs based on blood type antigens, the RH negative factor introduces specific considerations that warrant special attention. Here's why it's beneficial to focus on RH negative blood types:

1. Unique Nutritional Needs

Individuals with RH negative blood may have distinct nutritional requirements compared to those with RH positive blood. The absence of the RH antigen can influence how the body processes and responds to certain nutrients and foods. By focusing on RH negative blood types, we can tailor dietary recommendations to address these unique needs, potentially improving health outcomes and overall well-being.

2. Limited Research on RH Negative

While there is substantial research on blood type diets in general, the specific implications of RH negative blood are less explored. This gap presents an opportunity to delve deeper into how RH negative blood types interact with various foods and dietary patterns. By focusing on RH negative blood, we contribute to a more comprehensive understanding of how to optimize health for this particular group.

3. Addressing Health Concerns

RH negative individuals may experience specific health concerns that are influenced by their blood type. These concerns can include immune responses, digestive issues, and nutritional absorption. A tailored diet that considers the RH negative factor can help manage or mitigate these concerns, leading to better health management and enhanced quality of life.

4. Enhancing Personalization

The RH negative blood type adds another layer of personalization to dietary planning. While general dietary guidelines offer a broad approach, focusing on RH negative individuals allows for more precise recommendations. This personalization can lead to more effective dietary strategies that align with an individual's unique biological profile, potentially leading to greater health benefits.

5. Optimizing Performance and Well-Being

For those with RH negative blood, optimizing their diet according to their specific needs can lead to improvements in various aspects of health, including energy levels, mental clarity, and overall well-being. By understanding and addressing the unique requirements of RH negative blood types, individuals can achieve a more balanced and healthful lifestyle.

6. Bridging the Gap

Focusing on RH negative blood types helps bridge the gap between generalized dietary advice and personalized nutrition. While many dietary recommendations are based on broad principles, addressing the needs of RH negative individuals provides a more nuanced approach, allowing for better alignment of dietary practices with individual health profiles.

7. Providing Support and Guidance

Many people with RH negative blood types seek specific guidance to navigate their dietary choices effectively. By focusing on RH negative blood, we provide valuable resources and support tailored to their unique needs, empowering them to make informed decisions about their health and nutrition.

Focusing on RH negative blood types allows for a more personalized and precise approach to nutrition and health management. By addressing the unique needs, health concerns, and opportunities for optimization associated with RH negative blood, we can offer tailored recommendations that enhance overall well-being. This focus not only contributes to a deeper understanding of blood type-specific nutrition but also supports individuals in achieving their health goals more effectively.

Chapter 1: The RH Negative Diet Explained

2.1 The Role of Blood Type in Metabolism

Metabolism is the complex set of biochemical processes that occur within our bodies to maintain life, including the conversion of food into energy, the building and repair of tissues, and the elimination of waste. The concept that blood type can influence metabolism is based on the idea that the specific antigens present on red blood cells may affect how our bodies process nutrients and respond to different foods. Here's how blood type might play a role in metabolism:

1. Blood Type and Digestive Enzymes

One of the key areas where blood type may influence metabolism is through the production and activity of digestive enzymes. Digestive enzymes are crucial for breaking down proteins, fats, and carbohydrates into their component nutrients, which can then be absorbed and utilized by the body. Different blood types may have variations in enzyme activity, which could impact how efficiently certain foods are digested and metabolized.

For example:

- **Blood Type O:** Individuals with blood type O are often considered to have a robust digestive system that can handle higher levels of protein and fat. They may produce more efficient digestive enzymes for these macronutrients, making them well-suited to diets rich in animal proteins.
- **Blood Type A:** Those with blood type A may have different enzyme profiles, possibly favoring a diet higher in carbohydrates and plant-based proteins. Their digestive systems might process these nutrients differently compared to blood type O.

2. Food Compatibility and Nutrient Absorption

Blood type can also influence the body's ability to absorb and utilize specific nutrients. Some theories suggest that blood type antigens interact with dietary components in ways that affect nutrient absorption and utilization. For instance:

- **Lectins:** These are proteins found in various foods that can bind to blood type antigens. Certain lectins may affect how nutrients are absorbed or how foods are metabolized, potentially leading to differences in metabolic efficiency among different blood types.

3. Immune Response and Metabolism

The immune system plays a significant role in metabolism by affecting how the body responds to various foods and nutrients. Blood type antigens can influence immune responses, which in turn can impact metabolic processes. For example:

- **Inflammation:** Blood type-specific interactions with food components may influence inflammation levels in the body. Chronic inflammation can disrupt normal metabolic processes, leading to issues such as insulin resistance or metabolic syndrome.

4. Personalized Dietary Needs

Understanding the role of blood type in metabolism can help tailor dietary recommendations to better align with individual needs. Personalized nutrition based on blood type may enhance metabolic efficiency and overall health by focusing on foods and nutrients that are well-suited to the body's specific metabolic processes. For example:

- **Blood Type B:** Individuals with blood type B may benefit from a diet that includes a variety of foods, including dairy products and a mix of plant and animal proteins, due to their unique metabolic profile.

5. Scientific Evidence and Debate

While the idea that blood type influences metabolism is intriguing, it remains a topic of scientific debate. Some studies suggest that blood type-specific diets can lead to improvements in metabolic markers and overall health, while others find no significant differences compared to general dietary guidelines. More research is needed to fully understand the extent of these effects and to establish evidence-based recommendations.

The role of blood type in metabolism encompasses how digestive enzymes, nutrient absorption, immune responses, and overall metabolic efficiency may be influenced by blood type-specific factors. While there is evidence suggesting that blood type can impact these processes, the scientific community continues to explore and debate these interactions. By considering blood type in metabolic assessments and dietary planning, we can work towards more personalized and effective nutritional strategies to support individual health and well-being.

2.2 Key Principles of the RH Negative Diet

The RH Negative Diet is designed to optimize health by aligning dietary choices with the specific needs of individuals with RH negative blood types. Here are the key principles guiding this diet:

1. **Personalized Food Choices:** Focus on foods that are believed to be more compatible with RH negative blood types. This includes selecting nutrient-dense, easily digestible foods and avoiding those that may cause digestive issues or inflammation.
2. **Avoidance of Certain Foods:** Limit or avoid foods that are thought to interact negatively with RH negative blood, such as those containing problematic lectins or allergens. This includes certain grains, dairy products, and processed foods.
3. **Emphasis on Whole Foods:** Prioritize whole, unprocessed foods that are rich in essential nutrients. This includes lean proteins, fresh vegetables, fruits, nuts, and seeds.
4. **Balanced Nutrition:** Ensure a balanced intake of macronutrients (proteins, fats, and carbohydrates) and micronutrients (vitamins and minerals) tailored to the specific metabolic needs of RH negative individuals.
5. **Holistic Approach:** Integrate dietary choices with overall lifestyle factors, such as regular exercise, stress management, and adequate sleep, to support overall health and well-being.

By adhering to these principles, the RH Negative Diet aims to enhance metabolic function and overall health tailored to the unique needs of RH negative blood types.

2.3 Benefits of Following the RH Negative Diet

Following the RH Negative Diet offers several potential benefits tailored to the unique needs of individuals with RH negative blood types:

1. **Improved Digestive Health:** By focusing on foods that are compatible with RH negative blood types, individuals may experience better digestion and reduced gastrointestinal discomfort.
2. **Enhanced Nutrient Absorption:** The diet emphasizes nutrient-dense foods that support optimal absorption and utilization of essential vitamins and minerals.
3. **Reduced Inflammation:** Avoiding foods that may trigger inflammatory responses can lead to decreased inflammation and improved overall health.
4. **Increased Energy Levels:** A balanced diet aligned with RH negative needs can contribute to higher energy levels and improved overall vitality.
5. **Personalized Nutrition:** Tailoring dietary choices to blood type-specific needs can enhance metabolic efficiency and support individual health goals more effectively.

Chapter 2: Foods to Embrace

3.1 Ideal Foods for RH Negative Blood Types

For RH negative blood types, ideal foods include:

1. **Lean Proteins:** Opt for high-quality proteins such as lean meats (chicken, turkey), fish, and eggs, which support muscle health and energy levels.
2. **Fresh Vegetables:** Include a variety of vegetables like leafy greens (spinach, kale), broccoli, and bell peppers to provide essential vitamins and minerals.
3. **Fruits:** Focus on low-sugar fruits such as berries, apples, and pears for their antioxidant properties and nutritional benefits.
4. **Nuts and Seeds:** Incorporate nuts (almonds, walnuts) and seeds (chia, flax) for healthy fats and added nutrients.
5. **Whole Grains:** Select whole grains like quinoa and brown rice, which are more easily digestible and offer fiber and essential nutrients.

By prioritizing these foods, individuals with RH negative blood types can support optimal health and metabolic function.

3.2 Nutritional Benefits of These Foods

The ideal foods for RH negative blood types offer several nutritional benefits:

1. **Lean Proteins:** Provide essential amino acids for muscle repair and growth, support immune function, and help maintain steady energy levels.
2. **Fresh Vegetables:** Rich in vitamins (A, C, K), minerals (iron, calcium), and antioxidants that support immune health, reduce inflammation, and promote overall wellness.
3. **Fruits:** Offer antioxidants, vitamins, and fiber that help combat oxidative stress, support digestive health, and regulate blood sugar levels.
4. **Nuts and Seeds:** Supply healthy fats, protein, and essential nutrients like omega-3 fatty acids, which are beneficial for heart health and cognitive function.
5. **Whole Grains:** Deliver fiber, B vitamins, and minerals that aid in digestion, support sustained energy release, and contribute to cardiovascular health.

Incorporating these foods can enhance overall health and well-being by providing crucial nutrients and supporting the body's specific needs.

Chapter 3: Foods to Avoid

4.1 Foods That May Cause Issues for RH Negative Individuals

For RH negative individuals, certain foods may cause digestive or health issues due to their unique blood type characteristics:

1. **High-Lectin Foods:** Foods high in lectins, such as beans, lentils, and certain grains (like wheat and corn), may interfere with digestion and nutrient absorption by binding to blood type antigens.
2. **Dairy Products:** Some RH negative individuals may experience difficulties with dairy due to lactose intolerance or sensitivity, leading to gastrointestinal discomfort and inflammation.
3. **Processed Foods:** Foods high in additives, preservatives, and artificial ingredients can exacerbate inflammation and negatively impact overall health.
4. **Certain Meats:** Processed or high-fat meats may contribute to digestive issues or increase inflammation, affecting overall metabolic health.
5. **Refined Sugars and Carbohydrates:** High consumption of refined sugars and carbohydrates can lead to insulin resistance and metabolic imbalances, impacting overall health.

Avoiding or moderating these foods can help prevent potential health issues and promote better well-being for RH negative individuals.

4.2 Understanding Food Sensitivities and Reactions

Food sensitivities and reactions can significantly impact the health and well-being of individuals, particularly those with RH negative blood types. Understanding these sensitivities is crucial for managing and optimizing dietary choices:

1. Food Sensitivities: Food sensitivities occur when the digestive system reacts negatively to certain foods, leading to symptoms such as bloating, gas, or abdominal pain. For RH negative individuals, specific foods may trigger these sensitivities due to their interaction with blood type antigens or other metabolic factors.

2. Lectin Interactions: Lectins are proteins found in many foods that can bind to blood type antigens on the surface of cells. For RH negative individuals, certain lectins might cause gastrointestinal distress or interfere with nutrient absorption. This can lead to symptoms like cramping, diarrhea, or nausea.

3. Immune Reactions: Food sensitivities can also provoke immune responses, resulting in inflammation and other systemic reactions. RH negative individuals might be more prone to immune-related issues with certain foods, leading to symptoms such as fatigue, joint pain, or skin conditions.

4. Digestive Enzyme Activity: Variations in digestive enzyme activity can affect how well certain foods are broken down and absorbed. RH negative individuals may experience difficulties digesting specific foods, leading to discomfort or malabsorption issues.

5. Avoiding Trigger Foods: Identifying and avoiding foods that cause sensitivities or reactions is essential for maintaining optimal health. Keeping a food diary, monitoring symptoms, and working with a healthcare professional can help pinpoint problematic foods and tailor the diet accordingly.

By understanding and managing food sensitivities and reactions, RH negative individuals can make informed dietary choices that minimize discomfort and support overall well-being.

4.3 Alternatives and Substitutions

For RH negative individuals who need to avoid certain foods due to sensitivities or potential issues, finding suitable alternatives and substitutions can help maintain a balanced and enjoyable diet. Here are some effective alternatives and substitutions:

1. For High-Lectin Foods:

- **Legume Substitutes:** Replace beans and lentils with alternatives like quinoa, chia seeds, or hemp seeds, which are lower in lectins and still provide protein and fiber.
- **Grain Alternatives:** Opt for gluten-free grains such as rice, millet, or amaranth instead of wheat and corn.

2. For Dairy Products:

- **Non-Dairy Milks:** Use plant-based milks like almond, coconut, or oat milk as substitutes for cow's milk.
- **Dairy-Free Yogurts and Cheeses:** Explore options made from nuts or soy to replace traditional yogurt and cheese.

3. For Processed Foods:

- **Whole Food Snacks:** Choose snacks made from whole ingredients, such as fresh fruit, nuts, and seeds, instead of processed and packaged options.
- **Homemade Meals:** Prepare meals from scratch using fresh, whole ingredients to avoid additives and preservatives found in processed foods.

4. For Certain Meats:

- **Lean Proteins:** Substitute high-fat or processed meats with lean options like chicken breast, turkey, or fish.

- **Plant-Based Proteins:** Incorporate plant-based protein sources such as tofu, tempeh, or edamame for variety and to reduce reliance on red meat.

5. For Refined Sugars and Carbohydrates:

- **Natural Sweeteners:** Use natural sweeteners like honey, maple syrup, or stevia instead of refined sugars.
- **Whole Grains:** Replace refined carbohydrates with whole grains like brown rice, quinoa, or whole wheat alternatives for more fiber and nutrients.

By incorporating these alternatives and substitutions, RH negative individuals can create a diet that aligns with their health needs while avoiding problematic foods.

Chapter 4: Sample Meal Plans

5.1 7-Day Meal Plan for Beginners

This 7-day meal plan is designed for individuals with RH negative blood types who are new to the diet. It focuses on incorporating ideal foods while avoiding those that may cause issues. Each day features balanced meals to support overall health and well-being.

Day 1

- **Breakfast:** Scrambled eggs with spinach and tomatoes, served with a side of fresh berries.
- **Lunch:** Grilled chicken breast on a bed of mixed greens with cucumbers, bell peppers, and a vinaigrette dressing.
- **Dinner:** Baked salmon with roasted broccoli and quinoa.
- **Snack:** A handful of almonds.
- **Dessert:** Sliced apple with a drizzle of honey.

Day 2

- **Breakfast:** Smoothie with almond milk, banana, spinach, and chia seeds.
- **Lunch:** Turkey and avocado wrap in a gluten-free tortilla with a side of carrot sticks.
- **Dinner:** Stir-fried tofu with mixed vegetables (broccoli, bell peppers, snap peas) and brown rice.
- **Snack:** Celery sticks with almond butter.
- **Dessert:** Mixed berries with a dollop of coconut yogurt.

Day 3

- **Breakfast:** Oatmeal topped with fresh strawberries and a sprinkle of flaxseeds.

- **Lunch:** Quinoa salad with chickpeas, cucumbers, tomatoes, and a lemon-tahini dressing.
- **Dinner:** Grilled shrimp with a side of steamed asparagus and sweet potato mash.
- **Snack:** Apple slices with a handful of walnuts.
- **Dessert:** Baked pear with a touch of cinnamon.

Day 4

- **Breakfast:** Greek yogurt with blueberries and a sprinkle of chia seeds.
- **Lunch:** Chicken and vegetable soup with a side of mixed greens salad.
- **Dinner:** Beef stir-fry with bell peppers, onions, and snap peas over cauliflower rice.
- **Snack:** A small handful of pumpkin seeds.
- **Dessert:** Sliced kiwi and a handful of raspberries.

Day 5

- **Breakfast:** Smoothie bowl with almond milk, banana, spinach, and topped with sliced almonds and chia seeds.
- **Lunch:** Lentil and vegetable stew with a side of gluten-free bread.
- **Dinner:** Baked cod with roasted Brussels sprouts and a quinoa pilaf.
- **Snack:** Carrot sticks with hummus.
- **Dessert:** Chilled mango slices.

Day 6

- **Breakfast:** Avocado toast on gluten-free bread with a side of mixed fruit.
- **Lunch:** Grilled vegetable and quinoa salad with a balsamic vinaigrette.
- **Dinner:** Lemon herb roasted chicken thighs with a side of green beans and wild rice.
- **Snack:** A handful of cashews.
- **Dessert:** Chia pudding made with almond milk and topped with fresh strawberries.

Day 7

- **Breakfast:** Chia seed pudding with almond milk and topped with sliced bananas and a sprinkle of walnuts.
- **Lunch:** Spinach and chicken salad with avocado, cherry tomatoes, and a lemon-olive oil dressing.
- **Dinner:** Grilled tilapia with sautéed kale and sweet potato wedges.
- **Snack:** Fresh cucumber slices with a handful of sunflower seeds.
- **Dessert:** Fresh peach slices with a drizzle of honey.

This meal plan is designed to be simple and easy to follow, providing a variety of nutrient-dense foods while aligning with the principles of the RH Negative Diet. Adjust portions and ingredients as needed based on personal preferences and nutritional requirements.

5.2 Advanced Meal Planning for Long-Term Success

Advanced meal planning is key for maintaining adherence to the RH Negative Diet over the long term. It involves creating a structured and flexible approach to meals that supports sustained health and well-being. Here's how to implement an effective advanced meal planning strategy:

1. Establish Nutritional Goals:

- **Identify Personal Needs:** Determine your specific nutritional requirements based on your health goals, activity level, and any dietary restrictions. Consider consulting with a nutritionist or dietitian to tailor your plan.
- **Set Balanced Goals:** Aim for a balanced intake of macronutrients (proteins, fats, carbohydrates) and micronutrients (vitamins and minerals) to ensure comprehensive nutrition.

2. Create a Weekly Menu:

- **Diverse Meal Choices:** Plan a variety of meals each week to ensure a diverse intake of nutrients and prevent dietary monotony. Rotate different proteins, vegetables, and grains to keep meals interesting and balanced.
- **Include Make-Ahead Meals:** Incorporate recipes that can be prepared in advance and stored, such as soups, stews, and casseroles. This can save time and reduce meal prep stress during busy days.

3. Grocery Shopping and Batch Cooking:

- **Grocery Lists:** Create detailed grocery lists based on your weekly menu to streamline shopping and avoid impulse buys. Focus on whole, unprocessed foods that align with RH negative dietary needs.

- **Batch Cooking:** Prepare and cook larger quantities of staple items like grains, proteins, and vegetables. Store these in the refrigerator or freezer for quick and easy meal assembly throughout the week.

4. Flexible Meal Templates:

- **Meal Templates:** Develop meal templates that outline key components (protein, vegetable, grain) to simplify meal planning. For example, a template might include grilled protein, a vegetable stir-fry, and a whole grain side.
- **Adapt to Availability:** Be flexible with ingredient choices based on seasonal produce and availability. This helps maintain variety and freshness in your meals.

5. Monitor and Adjust:

- **Track Progress:** Regularly review your meal plan and track your health progress. Assess how well the diet aligns with your goals and make adjustments as needed.
- **Adjust Portions and Ingredients:** Modify portion sizes and ingredients based on changes in activity levels, health conditions, or personal preferences.

6. Incorporate Variety and Experimentation:

- **Try New Recipes:** Regularly introduce new recipes and cooking techniques to keep your diet engaging and prevent boredom. Experiment with different spices and herbs to add flavor without added salt or sugar.
- **Explore Alternatives:** Be open to exploring new food alternatives and substitutions that align with RH negative dietary guidelines.

7. Focus on Lifestyle Integration:

- **Meal Timing:** Consider incorporating strategies such as meal timing or intermittent fasting if they align with your goals and lifestyle.
- **Mindful Eating:** Practice mindful eating by focusing on portion sizes, eating slowly, and listening to your body's hunger and fullness cues.

8. Plan for Special Occasions:

- **Holiday and Event Planning:** Prepare for special occasions by planning ahead with suitable recipes and alternatives that fit your dietary needs. This helps you stay on track while enjoying social events.

By implementing these advanced meal planning strategies, you can achieve long-term success with the RH Negative Diet. This structured approach ensures that you maintain a balanced and varied diet, supports overall health, and fits seamlessly into your lifestyle.

Chapter 5: Recipes for Every Meal

6.1 Breakfast

6.1.1 Berry and Spinach Smoothie

Ingredients

- 1 cup fresh or frozen strawberries
- 1/2 cup blueberries
- 1/2 cup raspberries (optional)
- 2-3 cups spinach
- 1 banana
- 1/2 cup plain Greek yogurt or cottage cheese
- 1 cup unsweetened almond milk or soy milk

Directions

1. Add all ingredients to a blender in the order listed.
2. Blend on high speed until smooth and creamy, about 30-60 seconds.
3. Pour into a glass and enjoy immediately.

Prep Time

5 minutes

Serving Size

1 serving (makes about 2 cups)

Nutrition (per serving)

- Calories: 230-300 depending on ingredients
- Protein: 10-15g from yogurt/milk
- Fiber: 6-8g from fruits and veggies
- Vitamins A, C, K, folate, manganese, magnesium from spinach
- Antioxidants from berries

6.1.2 Quinoa Breakfast Bowl

Ingredients

- 1 cup uncooked quinoa
- 1 cup water (for cooking quinoa)
- 1/2 avocado, sliced
- 1 cup cooked black beans
- 3 tomatoes, diced
- 1/2 white onion, chopped
- 1-2 jalapeños, diced (optional)
- 1 cup chopped cilantro
- 2 eggs (fried or hard-boiled)
- 1-2 limes (for juice)
- Sea salt to taste
- Spicy salsa (for serving)

Directions

1. **Cook the Quinoa**: Rinse the quinoa under cold water. In a saucepan, combine the rinsed quinoa and water. Bring to a boil, then reduce heat to low, cover, and simmer for about 15 minutes until the quinoa is fluffy and the water is absorbed. Alternatively, you can use an Instant Pot, cooking it on high pressure for 1 minute and allowing for natural pressure release.
2. **Prepare the Pico de Gallo**: While the quinoa is cooking, chop the onion, tomatoes, cilantro, and jalapeños. Combine them in a bowl, adding lime juice and sea salt to taste.
3. **Cook the Eggs**: If using fried eggs, cook them in a skillet to your liking. For hard-boiled eggs, you can add them to the Instant Pot with the quinoa.
4. **Assemble the Bowl**: In two bowls, layer the cooked quinoa, black beans, pico de gallo, sliced avocado, and the cooked eggs. Drizzle with spicy salsa and additional lime juice if desired.

Prep Time

10 minutes

Cook Time

15-20 minutes (depending on cooking method for quinoa and eggs)

Serving Size

Serves 2

Nutrition (per serving)

- Calories: Approximately 400-500 (varies based on toppings)
- Protein: 20-25g (from quinoa, beans, and eggs)
- Fiber: 10-12g (from quinoa, beans, and vegetables)
- Healthy fats: 15-20g (from avocado)
- Vitamins and minerals: Rich in vitamins A, C, K, folate, and iron from the vegetables and quinoa.

6.1.3 Avocado and Egg Toast

Ingredients

- 1 slice whole grain or sourdough bread, toasted
- 1/2 ripe avocado
- 1 large egg (cooked to your preference: fried, poached, scrambled, or hard-boiled)
- Sea salt, to taste
- Freshly cracked black pepper, to taste
- Optional: hot sauce or red pepper flakes, for added flavor
- Optional: a squeeze of lemon juice or olive oil for drizzling

Directions

1. **Toast the Bread**: Start by toasting your slice of bread until golden brown and crispy.
2. **Prepare the Avocado**: While the bread is toasting, cut the avocado in half, remove the pit, and scoop the flesh into a bowl. Mash it with a fork, adding a pinch of salt and pepper, and a squeeze of lemon juice if desired.
3. **Cook the Egg**: Prepare the egg according to your preference:
   - **Fried**: Heat a small nonstick skillet over medium heat, add a little butter or oil, crack the egg into the skillet, and cook until the whites are set and the yolk is to your liking (about 5-7 minutes).
   - **Poached**: Bring a pot of water to a gentle simmer, add a splash of vinegar, create a vortex with a spoon, and gently drop in the egg. Cook for 3-4 minutes.
   - **Scrambled**: Whisk the egg in a bowl, pour into a heated skillet, and gently stir until cooked through (about 2-3 minutes).
   - **Hard-boiled**: Place eggs in boiling water for 9-12 minutes, then cool in ice water before peeling.

4. **Assemble the Toast**: Spread the mashed avocado generously over the toasted bread. Top with the cooked egg.

5. **Season and Serve**: Sprinkle with additional salt and pepper, and add hot sauce or red pepper flakes if desired. Enjoy immediately.

Prep Time

5 minutes

Cook Time

5-10 minutes (depending on the egg cooking method)

Serving Size

1 serving

Nutrition (per serving)

- Calories: Approximately 250-300 (varies based on ingredients and cooking method)
- Protein: 10-15g (from the egg)
- Healthy Fats: 15-20g (from the avocado)
- Carbohydrates: 20-30g (from the bread)
- Fiber: 6-8g (from the avocado and whole grain bread)

6.1.4 Greek Yogurt with Nuts and Honey

Ingredients

- 2 cups full-fat Greek yogurt
- 1/2 cup high-quality honey (preferably organic)
- 1 cup walnuts (toasted)
- 3/4 teaspoon vanilla extract (optional)
- Cinnamon powder (optional, for garnish)

Directions

1. **Toast the Walnuts**: Preheat your oven to 350°F (180°C). Spread the walnuts in a single layer on a baking sheet and toast for 5-6 minutes, or until golden and fragrant. Allow them to cool.
2. **Prepare the Yogurt**: In a bowl, mix the Greek yogurt with vanilla extract if using. This step adds extra flavor but can be skipped if you prefer a simpler taste.
3. **Assemble the Dish**: In serving bowls, add a generous portion of the yogurt. Drizzle with honey and top with the toasted walnuts.
4. **Garnish**: If desired, sprinkle with cinnamon powder for added flavor.
5. **Serve**: Enjoy immediately as a breakfast, snack, or dessert.

Prep Time

5 minutes

Cook Time

5-6 minutes (for toasting walnuts)

Serving Size

Serves 2-4, depending on portion size

Nutrition (per serving, based on 2 servings)

- Calories: Approximately 400-450 kcal
- Protein: 15-20g (from yogurt)
- Fat: 20-25g (from walnuts and yogurt)

- Carbohydrates: 40-50g (from honey)
- Fiber: 2-3g (from walnuts)
- Sugar: 30-35g (from honey)

6.1.5 Sweet Potato Hash

Ingredients

- 2 large sweet potatoes, cut into 1/2-inch cubes
- 1/2 medium red onion, chopped
- 1 poblano pepper, stemmed, seeded, and chopped (or bell pepper)
- 2 garlic cloves, thinly sliced
- 4 teaspoons avocado oil (or olive oil)
- 1 teaspoon chili powder
- 4 leaves lacinato kale, stemmed and torn (optional)
- 4 large eggs (optional)
- Sea salt and freshly ground black pepper, to taste
- Optional toppings: sliced avocado, fresh cilantro, hot sauce, lime wedges

Directions

1. **Prepare the Vegetables**: In a large skillet, heat the avocado oil over medium heat. Add the chopped onion and poblano pepper, cooking until softened, about 5 minutes. Add the sliced garlic and cook for an additional minute.
2. **Cook the Sweet Potatoes**: Add the sweet potato cubes to the skillet. Season with salt, pepper, and chili powder. Stir well to combine. Cover the skillet and cook for about 10-15 minutes, stirring occasionally, until the sweet potatoes are tender.
3. **Add Kale (Optional)**: If using kale, stir it into the mixture and cook for another 2-3 minutes until wilted.
4. **Cook the Eggs (Optional)**: If you want to add eggs, create four wells in the hash and crack an egg into each well. Cover the skillet and cook for 3-5 minutes until the eggs are set to your liking.
5. **Serve**: Remove from heat and serve hot, topped with avocado slices, fresh cilantro, hot sauce, and lime wedges if desired.

Prep Time

10 minutes

Cook Time

20-25 minutes

Serving Size

Serves 4

Nutrition (per serving, without eggs)

- Calories: Approximately 250-300 kcal
- Protein: 5-7g (from sweet potatoes and vegetables)
- Fat: 10-15g (from oil)
- Carbohydrates: 40-45g (from sweet potatoes)
- Fiber: 6-8g (from sweet potatoes and vegetables)
- Sugar: 5-7g (naturally occurring in sweet potatoes)

6.1.6 Chia Pudding with Almond Milk

Ingredients

- 2 tablespoons chia seeds
- 1/2 to 2/3 cup unsweetened almond milk (adjust for desired consistency)
- 1 tablespoon maple syrup or honey (adjust to taste)
- Pinch of salt (optional)
- 1/4 teaspoon vanilla extract (optional)
- Optional toppings: fresh fruit, nuts, granola, or coconut flakes

Directions

1. **Combine Ingredients**: In a medium bowl or a mason jar, whisk together the chia seeds, almond milk, maple syrup (or honey), and vanilla extract if using.
2. **Initial Stir**: Stir the mixture well to ensure there are no clumps of chia seeds.
3. **Let It Sit**: Allow the mixture to sit for about 5 minutes, then stir again to break up any lumps that may have formed.
4. **Refrigerate**: Cover the bowl or jar and refrigerate for at least 2 hours, or ideally overnight. This allows the chia seeds to absorb the liquid and thicken into a pudding-like consistency.
5. **Serve**: When ready to eat, give the pudding a good stir and top with your choice of fresh fruit, nuts, granola, or coconut flakes before serving.

Prep Time

5 minutes

Soaking Time

2 hours (or overnight for best results)

Serving Size

Serves 1-2, depending on portion size

Nutrition (per serving, based on 1/2 cup almond milk)

- Calories: Approximately 150-200 kcal

- Protein: 4-5g (from chia seeds)
- Fat: 7-10g (from chia seeds and almond milk)
- Carbohydrates: 15-20g (mainly from almond milk and sweetener)
- Fiber: 10g (from chia seeds)
- Sugar: 5-10g (depends on sweetener used)

6.1.7 Oatmeal with Apple and Cinnamon

Ingredients

- 1 cup old-fashioned rolled oats
- 2 cups water or milk (or a combination)
- 1 medium apple, cored and chopped (e.g., Honeycrisp, Granny Smith)
- 1/2 teaspoon ground cinnamon
- 1 tablespoon maple syrup or honey (optional, adjust to taste)
- Pinch of salt
- Optional toppings: chopped nuts (e.g., walnuts or pecans), additional apple slices, raisins, or a dollop of yogurt

Directions

1. **Cook the Oats**: In a medium saucepan, bring the water (or milk) to a boil. Stir in the oats and a pinch of salt. Reduce heat to low and simmer for about 5-7 minutes, stirring occasionally, until the oats are tender and have absorbed most of the liquid.
2. **Prepare the Apples**: While the oats are cooking, in a separate small skillet, add a little water or a small amount of butter. Add the chopped apple and sauté over medium heat for about 3-5 minutes until they are softened. Sprinkle the cinnamon over the apples and stir to combine.
3. **Combine**: Once the oats are cooked, stir in the sautéed apples and maple syrup or honey if using. Mix well to combine all ingredients.
4. **Serve**: Spoon the oatmeal into bowls and top with your choice of nuts, additional apple slices, or raisins. Drizzle with more maple syrup if desired.

Prep Time

5 minutes

Cook Time

10 minutes

Serving Size

Serves 2

Nutrition (per serving)

- Calories: Approximately 250-300 kcal
- Protein: 6-8g (from oats and optional toppings)
- Fat: 4-6g (depends on added nuts or butter)
- Carbohydrates: 45-50g (mainly from oats and apples)
- Fiber: 6-8g (from oats and apples)
- Sugar: 10-15g (natural sugars from apples and sweetener)

6.1.8 Veggie Omelette

Ingredients

- 3 large eggs
- 2 teaspoons milk, cream, or sour cream
- 1 tablespoon butter, divided
- 1/4 cup chopped mushrooms
- 2 tablespoons finely chopped white onion
- 2 tablespoons finely chopped green bell pepper
- 2 tablespoons finely chopped red bell pepper
- 2 tablespoons shredded cheddar cheese
- Salt and pepper to taste

Directions

1. **Beat the eggs and dairy**: In a small bowl, whisk together the eggs and milk (or cream/sour cream) until smooth and well combined.
2. **Sauté the veggies**: In a large sauté pan, melt half of the butter over medium heat. Add the mushrooms, onion, green and red bell peppers. Cook until softened, about 5-7 minutes.
3. **Cook the eggs**: Melt the remaining butter in the pan. Reduce heat to medium-low and pour in the egg mixture. Allow the bottom to set slightly, about 2-3 minutes.
4. **Fold the omelette**: When the egg is almost fully cooked, sprinkle the shredded cheese over one half of the omelette. Fold the unfilled half over the cheese half.
5. **Finish cooking**: Allow the omelette to cook for another minute or until the cheese is melted and the egg is set.
6. **Serve**: Slide the folded omelette onto a plate. Season with salt and pepper to taste. Serve immediately.

Prep Time

5 minutes

Cook Time

10 minutes

Serving Size

1 omelette

Nutrition (per serving)

- Calories: 358
- Protein: 22g
- Fat: 27g
- Carbohydrates: 8g
- Fiber: 2g
- Sugar: 3g

6.1.9 Smoothie Bowl with Toppings

Ingredients

For the Smoothie Base:

- 1 cup frozen mixed berries (such as strawberries, blueberries, raspberries)
- 1 frozen banana, sliced
- 1/2 cup unsweetened almond milk
- 1 tablespoon almond butter
- 1 tablespoon honey (optional)

Toppings:

- 1/4 cup granola
- 2 tablespoons sliced almonds
- 2 tablespoons unsweetened shredded coconut
- 1 tablespoon chia seeds
- Fresh berries (such as blueberries, raspberries, sliced strawberries)

Directions

1. **Make the Smoothie Base**: In a high-speed blender, combine the frozen mixed berries, frozen banana slices, almond milk, almond butter, and honey (if using). Blend until smooth and creamy, adding more almond milk as needed to reach desired consistency.
2. **Pour the Smoothie**: Transfer the smoothie to a bowl.
3. **Add the Toppings**: Sprinkle the granola, sliced almonds, shredded coconut, and chia seeds over the smoothie. Top with fresh berries.
4. **Serve Immediately**: Enjoy the smoothie bowl right away with a spoon.

Prep Time

5 minutes

Cook Time

None

Serving Size

1 bowl

Nutrition (per serving)

- Calories: 450
- Protein: 10g
- Fat: 20g
- Carbohydrates: 60g
- Fiber: 12g
- Sugar: 35g

6.1.10 Coconut Flour Pancakes

Ingredients

- 1/3 cup coconut flour
- 1 teaspoon baking powder
- 2 large eggs
- 1/3 cup unsweetened almond milk (or any milk of choice)
- 1 teaspoon vanilla extract
- 1 tablespoon maple syrup (optional)
- Pinch of salt
- Optional toppings: fresh fruit, nut butter, maple syrup, or shredded coconut

Directions

1. **Mix Dry Ingredients**: In a large bowl, combine the coconut flour, baking powder, and salt. Whisk together until well blended.
2. **Mix Wet Ingredients**: In a separate bowl, whisk together the eggs, almond milk, maple syrup (if using), and vanilla extract.
3. **Combine Mixtures**: Pour the wet ingredients into the dry ingredients and stir until just combined. Let the batter sit for 2-3 minutes to allow the coconut flour to absorb the liquid.
4. **Cook the Pancakes**: Heat a non-stick skillet or griddle over medium heat and lightly grease it with butter or oil. Pour about 1/4 cup of batter for each pancake onto the skillet. Cook for 2-3 minutes, or until bubbles form on the surface and the edges look set. Flip and cook for another 2-3 minutes until golden brown.
5. **Serve**: Remove from the skillet and serve warm with your choice of toppings.

Prep Time

5 minutes

Cook Time

10 minutes

Serving Size

Serves 2-3 (approximately 4-6 pancakes)

Nutrition (per serving, based on 2 servings)

- Calories: Approximately 250-300 kcal
- Protein: 12-15g
- Fat: 14-16g
- Carbohydrates: 30g
- Fiber: 10g
- Sugar: 2-5g (depending on optional ingredients)

6.1.11 Egg and Veggie Breakfast Muffins

Ingredients

- 6 large eggs
- 1 cup egg whites (or an additional 6 eggs)
- 1/2 teaspoon sea salt
- 1/2 teaspoon ground black pepper
- 1 teaspoon olive oil
- 1/2 orange bell pepper, chopped
- 1/2 cup yellow onion, chopped
- 1 cup broccoli, chopped into small pieces
- 1 cup mushrooms, sliced
- 1/3 cup crumbled feta cheese (optional)
- 2 tablespoons fresh parsley, chopped (optional)
- Cooking spray (for muffin tin)

Directions

1. **Preheat the Oven**: Preheat your oven to 375°F (190°C). Spray a 12-cup muffin tin with cooking spray or line with silicone baking cups.
2. **Sauté the Vegetables**: In a skillet, heat the olive oil over medium heat. Add the chopped bell pepper, onion, broccoli, and mushrooms. Sauté for about 5-6 minutes until the vegetables are softened and the onions are fragrant.
3. **Whisk the Eggs**: In a large bowl, whisk together the eggs, egg whites, salt, and pepper until well combined.
4. **Combine Ingredients**: Add the sautéed vegetables to the egg mixture. If using, stir in the crumbled feta cheese and fresh parsley.
5. **Fill Muffin Cups**: Pour the egg and vegetable mixture evenly into the prepared muffin cups, filling each about 2/3 full.
6. **Bake**: Bake in the preheated oven for 17-20 minutes, or until the egg muffins are set and a toothpick inserted in the center comes out clean.

7. **Cool and Serve**: Allow the muffins to cool slightly before removing them from the tin. Serve warm or store in an airtight container in the refrigerator for up to 4 days.

Prep Time

10 minutes

Cook Time

20 minutes

Serving Size

Serves 6 (2 muffins per serving)

Nutrition (per muffin, based on 12 muffins)

- Calories: Approximately 75-100 kcal
- Protein: 7g
- Fat: 5g
- Carbohydrates: 2g
- Fiber: 1g
- Sugar: 1g

6.1.12 Buckwheat Porridge

Ingredients

- 1 cup raw buckwheat groats
- 3 cups water or non-dairy milk (such as almond or coconut milk)
- 1/4 teaspoon kosher salt
- Optional add-ins:
    - 1 tablespoon maple syrup or honey (for sweetness)
    - 1/2 teaspoon cinnamon (for flavor)
    - Fresh fruit (such as berries or sliced bananas)
    - Chia seeds or hemp seeds (for added nutrition)

Directions

1. **Rinse the Buckwheat**: Place the buckwheat groats in a fine mesh strainer and rinse them thoroughly under cold water to remove any dust or impurities.
2. **Cook the Buckwheat**: In a medium saucepan, combine the rinsed buckwheat groats, water (or non-dairy milk), and salt. Bring to a boil over medium-high heat.
3. **Simmer**: Once boiling, reduce the heat to low, cover, and let it simmer for about 10 minutes, stirring occasionally to prevent sticking.
4. **Let It Rest**: After 10 minutes, remove the saucepan from heat and let it sit, covered, for an additional 5 minutes. This allows the buckwheat to absorb any remaining liquid.
5. **Add Flavor**: Stir in any optional add-ins like maple syrup, cinnamon, or chia seeds. Mix well.
6. **Serve**: Ladle the porridge into bowls and top with fresh fruit, nuts, or any toppings of your choice. Enjoy warm.

Prep Time

5 minutes

Cook Time

15 minutes

Serving Size

Serves 4

Nutrition (per serving)

- Calories: Approximately 266 kcal
- Protein: 10g
- Fat: 2g
- Carbohydrates: 54g
- Fiber: 7g
- Sugar: 2g (without added sweeteners)

6.1.13 Pumpkin Spice Smoothie

Ingredients

- 1/2 cup canned pumpkin puree (not pie filling)
- 1 frozen banana, sliced
- 1/2 cup unsweetened almond milk (or milk of choice)
- 1/3 cup plain Greek yogurt
- 1-2 tablespoons maple syrup or honey (to taste)
- 1 teaspoon pumpkin pie spice
- 1/2 teaspoon vanilla extract
- Pinch of cinnamon
- 1/2 cup ice cubes

Directions

1. Add all the ingredients to a blender in the order listed.
2. Blend on high speed until smooth and creamy, about 30-60 seconds.
3. Pour into a glass and enjoy immediately.

Prep Time

5 minutes

Serving Size

1 serving (makes about 16 oz)

Nutrition (per serving)

- Calories: 250-300
- Protein: 10-15g (from yogurt)
- Fiber: 5-7g (from pumpkin and banana)
- Vitamin A: Over 100% DV from pumpkin
- Potassium: Good source from banana and pumpkin
- Calcium: From yogurt

6.1.14 Almond Flour Waffles

Ingredients

- 2 cups fine blanched almond flour
- 3 large eggs
- ½ cup unsweetened almond milk (or any milk of choice)
- 2 tablespoons melted coconut oil or avocado oil
- 1 tablespoon maple syrup (optional)
- 2 teaspoons baking powder
- 1 teaspoon vanilla extract
- 1 teaspoon cinnamon (optional)
- ½ teaspoon sea salt
- Cooking spray (for the waffle iron)
- Optional toppings: maple syrup, fresh berries, nut butter, or sliced bananas

Directions

1. **Preheat the Waffle Iron**: Preheat your waffle iron to medium-high heat and spray with cooking spray.
2. **Mix Wet Ingredients**: In a medium mixing bowl, whisk together the eggs, almond milk, melted coconut oil, maple syrup (if using), and vanilla extract until well combined.
3. **Combine Dry Ingredients**: In another bowl, mix together the almond flour, baking powder, cinnamon (if using), and sea salt.
4. **Combine Mixtures**: Pour the dry ingredients into the wet ingredients and stir until just combined. Let the batter sit for about 5 minutes to thicken.
5. **Cook the Waffles**: Pour about ½ cup of the batter onto the preheated waffle iron. Close the lid and cook for about 3-4 minutes, or until the waffles are golden brown and the iron stops steaming.
6. **Serve**: Carefully remove the waffles from the iron and serve immediately with your choice of toppings.

Prep Time

10 minutes

Cook Time

15 minutes

Serving Size

Serves 4 (approximately 4 waffles)

Nutrition (per waffle)

- Calories: 375 kcal
- Protein: 13g
- Fat: 29g
- Carbohydrates: 13g
- Fiber: 6g
- Sugar: 6g

6.1.15 Smoked Salmon and Avocado Wrap

Ingredients

- 2 tortilla wraps (can be gluten-free)
- 2 slices of oak-smoked smoked salmon
- 1 avocado, mashed
- 1 tablespoon mayonnaise
- 1 tablespoon chopped dill
- 1 tablespoon Dijon mustard
- 1 small carrot, shredded
- 4 large lettuce leaves
- Lemon juice
- Salt and pepper to taste

Directions

1. In a bowl, mix together the mashed avocado, dill, mayonnaise, mustard, lemon juice, salt and pepper until well combined.
2. Lay a tortilla wrap on a flat surface and spread the avocado mixture over it.
3. Top with the smoked salmon slices, shredded carrot and lettuce leaves.
4. Roll up the wrap tightly and cut in half diagonally to serve.

Prep Time

5 minutes

Cook Time

None

Serving Size

1 wrap

Nutrition (per serving)

- Calories: 498
- Protein: 43.6g

- Fat: 19.8g
- Carbohydrates: 30.1g
- Fiber: 10.9g
- Sodium: 346mg

6.2 Lunch

6.2.1 Quinoa and Black Bean Salad

Ingredients

For the Salad:

- 1 cup dry quinoa (yields about 3 cups cooked)
- 1 (15 oz) can black beans, drained and rinsed
- 2 cups cherry tomatoes, quartered
- 1 cup bell pepper (red or orange), finely diced
- 1/2 cup red onion, finely chopped
- 1 cup corn kernels (fresh or frozen)
- 1/2 cup fresh cilantro, chopped
- 1 medium avocado, diced (optional)

For the Dressing:

- 1/4 cup extra virgin olive oil
- 1/4 cup freshly squeezed lime juice
- 1 tablespoon apple cider vinegar
- 1 tablespoon maple syrup (or honey)
- 1 clove garlic, minced
- 1 teaspoon ground cumin
- 1/8 teaspoon cayenne pepper (optional)
- Salt to taste

Directions

1. **Cook the Quinoa:**
   - Rinse 1 cup of dry quinoa under cold water.
   - In a saucepan, combine the rinsed quinoa and 2 cups of water.

- ○ Bring to a boil, then reduce heat to low, cover, and simmer for about 15 minutes until the water is absorbed.
  - ○ Remove from heat and let sit, covered, for 5 minutes. Fluff with a fork and let cool.

2. **Prepare the Dressing:**
   - ○ In a bowl, whisk together the olive oil, lime juice, apple cider vinegar, maple syrup, minced garlic, cumin, cayenne pepper (if using), and salt.
3. **Combine the Salad:**
   - ○ In a large bowl, add the cooled quinoa, black beans, cherry tomatoes, bell pepper, red onion, corn, and cilantro.
   - ○ Pour the dressing over the salad and mix well to combine.
4. **Chill and Serve:**
   - ○ Refrigerate the salad for at least 1 hour before serving.
   - ○ If using, add diced avocado just before serving.

Cooking and Prep Time

- **Prep Time:** 15 minutes
- **Cook Time:** 15 minutes
- **Total Time:** 30 minutes (plus chilling time)

Serving

- Serves approximately 4-6 as a side dish or 2-4 as a main dish.

Nutritional Information (per serving, based on 6 servings)

- **Calories:** 206
- **Carbohydrates:** 22g
- **Protein:** 8g
- **Fat:** 11g
- **Saturated Fat:** 1.5g
- **Sodium:** 65mg

- **Potassium:** 333mg
- **Fiber:** 4g
- **Sugar:** 4g

6.2.2 Grilled Chicken and Veggie Wrap

Ingredients

- **Chicken**: 8 grilled chicken thighs (or 12 ounces boneless, skinless chicken breasts)
- **Tortillas**: 4 large whole wheat or gluten-free tortillas
- **Vegetables**:
    - 1 yellow sweet pepper (or red/orange)
    - 1 medium red bell pepper (optional)
    - 1 cup baby spinach leaves (or arugula)
    - 1/2 zucchini, cut into strips (optional)
-
- **Cream Cheese**: 4 tablespoons herb and garlic cream cheese (or any cheese of your choice)
- **Avocado**: 1 avocado, sliced (optional)
- **Hot Sauce**: 1 tablespoon (optional)
- **Olive Oil**: For drizzling
- **Seasonings**: Salt and pepper to taste

Directions

1. **Prep the Chicken**: If using raw chicken, grill or bake it until fully cooked. Slice into 1/2 inch strips.
2. **Prepare the Vegetables**: Slice the yellow and red peppers, zucchini, and avocado into strips.
3. **Warm the Tortillas**: Heat a skillet or non-stick pan over medium heat. Optionally, warm the tortillas in the oven for a few minutes.
4. **Assemble the Wraps**:
    - Spread 1 tablespoon of cream cheese on the bottom third of each tortilla.
    - Layer 1/4 cup of baby spinach over the cream cheese.
    - Add the sliced chicken, followed by the pepper strips and avocado slices.

    ○ Drizzle with hot sauce if desired.

5. **Wrap It Up**: Fold the sides of the tortilla towards the center, then roll from the bottom up to form a wrap.

6. **Cook the Wraps**: Place the wrapped tortilla seam-side down in the skillet. Cook until golden brown on all sides, about 2-3 minutes per side.

7. **Serve**: Cut the wraps in half and serve warm, optionally with a side of pickles or cornichons.

Cooking and Prep Time

- **Prep Time**: 15 minutes
- **Cooking Time**: 5-10 minutes
- **Total Time**: 20-25 minutes
- **Servings**: 4 wraps

Nutrition Information (per serving)

- **Calories**: Approximately 300 kcal
- **Total Fat**: 9 g
- **Saturated Fat**: 2.5 g
- **Cholesterol**: 75 mg
- **Sodium**: 540 mg
- **Total Carbohydrates**: 22 g
- **Dietary Fiber**: 5 g
- **Sugars**: 4 g
- **Protein**: 30 g
- **Vitamin A**: 40% DV
- **Vitamin C**: 60% DV
- **Calcium**: 10% DV
- **Iron**: 10% DV

6.2.3 Mediterranean Chickpea Salad

Ingredients

- 2 (15-ounce) cans chickpeas, drained and rinsed
- 1 large cucumber, diced
- 1 red bell pepper, diced
- 2 cups cherry tomatoes, halved
- 1/2 cup chopped roasted red peppers
- 1/4 cup diced red onion
- 4 ounces crumbled feta cheese
- 1/4 cup chopped fresh parsley
- 2 tablespoons extra-virgin olive oil
- 2 tablespoons lemon juice
- 1 garlic clove, minced
- 3/4 teaspoon sea salt
- Freshly ground black pepper

Instructions

1. In a large bowl, whisk together the olive oil, lemon juice, garlic, salt, and black pepper to make the dressing.
2. Add the chickpeas, cucumber, bell pepper, tomatoes, roasted red peppers, onion, and parsley to the bowl. Toss to coat with the dressing.
3. Transfer the salad to a serving platter. Top with crumbled feta cheese.

Cooking and Prep Time

- Prep Time: 15-20 minutes
- Total Time: 15-20 minutes

Serving and Nutrition

- Servings: 4-6
- Calories: Approximately 300 per serving

- Carbohydrates: 34g
- Protein: 12g
- Fat: 14g
- Fiber: 9g

6.2.4 Sweet Potato and Kale Salad

Ingredients

- 2 medium sweet potatoes, peeled and diced into 1/2-inch cubes (about 3 cups)
- 2 tablespoons olive oil, divided
- 1 teaspoon salt, divided
- 1/2 teaspoon black pepper, divided
- 1 bunch kale, stems removed and leaves thinly sliced (about 4 cups)
- 1/4 cup crumbled feta cheese
- 1/4 cup toasted pumpkin seeds or sunflower seeds
- 2 tablespoons dried cranberries or cherries
- For the Dressing:
    - 2 tablespoons olive oil
    - 2 tablespoons balsamic vinegar
    - 1 tablespoon honey
    - 1 garlic clove, minced
    - 1/4 teaspoon dried oregano
    - Salt and pepper to taste

Instructions

1. **Preheat** the oven to 400°F. Line a baking sheet with parchment paper.
2. **In a large bowl**, toss the diced sweet potatoes with 1 tablespoon olive oil, 1/2 teaspoon salt, and 1/4 teaspoon black pepper. Spread in a single layer on the prepared baking sheet.
3. **Roast** for 20-25 minutes, flipping halfway, until the sweet potatoes are tender and lightly browned. Allow to cool slightly.
4. **In a small bowl**, whisk together the dressing ingredients: olive oil, balsamic vinegar, honey, garlic, oregano, and the remaining 1/2 teaspoon salt and 1/4 teaspoon black pepper.

5. **Add** the sliced kale to a large bowl. Drizzle with the remaining 1 tablespoon olive oil and a pinch of salt. Massage the kale with your hands for 1-2 minutes until softened.

6. **Add** the roasted sweet potatoes, feta, seeds, and dried cranberries to the kale. Pour the dressing over top and toss to coat evenly.

7. **Serve** immediately or refrigerate until ready to serve. The salad will keep well for up to 4 days in the fridge.

Cooking and Prep Time

- Prep Time: 15 minutes
- Cook Time: 25 minutes
- Total Time: 40 minutes

Serving and Nutrition

- Servings: 4-6
- Calories: Approximately 300 per serving
- Carbohydrates: 35g
- Protein: 6g
- Fat: 16g
- Fiber: 6g

6.2.5 Lentil Soup

Ingredients

- ¼ cup extra virgin olive oil
- 1 medium yellow or white onion, chopped
- 2 carrots, peeled and chopped
- 4 garlic cloves, pressed or minced
- 2 teaspoons ground cumin
- 1 teaspoon curry powder
- ½ teaspoon dried thyme
- 1 (28-ounce) can diced tomatoes, lightly drained
- 1 cup brown or green lentils, picked over and rinsed
- 4 cups vegetable broth
- 2 cups water
- 1 teaspoon salt (more to taste)
- Pinch of red pepper flakes
- Freshly ground black pepper, to taste
- 1 cup chopped fresh kale or collard greens, tough ribs removed
- 1 to 2 tablespoons lemon juice (½ to 1 medium lemon), to taste

Directions

1. **Heat the Oil**: In a large Dutch oven or pot, warm the olive oil over medium heat until shimmering.
2. **Sauté Vegetables**: Add the chopped onion and carrots to the pot. Cook, stirring often, until the onion is softened and translucent, about 5 minutes.
3. **Add Spices and Garlic**: Stir in the minced garlic, cumin, curry powder, and thyme. Cook for about 30 seconds until fragrant.
4. **Incorporate Tomatoes and Lentils**: Pour in the drained diced tomatoes and cook for a few more minutes. Then add the lentils, vegetable broth, water, salt, and red pepper flakes. Season generously with black pepper.

5. **Simmer**: Raise the heat to bring the mixture to a boil. Once boiling, partially cover the pot and reduce the heat to maintain a gentle simmer. Cook for 25-30 minutes, or until the lentils are tender but still hold their shape.

6. **Blend (Optional)**: For a creamier texture, transfer 2 cups of the soup to a blender and purée until smooth. Return the puréed soup to the pot. Alternatively, use an immersion blender to blend a portion of the soup.

7. **Add Greens**: Stir in the chopped greens and cook for an additional 5 minutes, or until the greens are tender.

8. **Finish and Serve**: Remove from heat and stir in lemon juice. Taste and adjust seasoning with more salt, pepper, or lemon juice as desired. Serve hot.

Cooking and Prep Time

- **Prep Time**: 10 minutes
- **Cook Time**: 45 minutes
- **Total Time**: 55 minutes
- **Servings**: 4-6

Nutrition Information (per serving)

- **Calories**: Approximately 300 kcal
- **Total Fat**: 10 g
- **Saturated Fat**: 1.5 g
- **Cholesterol**: 0 mg
- **Sodium**: 600 mg
- **Total Carbohydrates**: 40 g
- **Dietary Fiber**: 15 g
- **Sugars**: 5 g
- **Protein**: 15 g

6.2.6 Turkey and Avocado Lettuce Wraps

Ingredients

- **For the Filling**:
    - 1 tablespoon olive oil
    - 1 large yellow onion, chopped
    - 1 lb lean ground turkey
    - 1 tablespoon chili powder
    - 1 teaspoon ground cumin
    - 1 teaspoon salt
    - 1/2 teaspoon black pepper
    - 1 avocado, diced
    - 1 tablespoon lime juice
    - 1 head of butter or romaine lettuce, leaves separated

- **For Serving**:
    - Fresh cilantro, chopped (optional)
    - Lime wedges (optional)

Directions

1. **Cook the Turkey**: In a large skillet, heat the olive oil over medium heat. Add the chopped onion and sauté until softened, about 5 minutes.
2. **Add Ground Turkey**: Stir in the ground turkey, chili powder, cumin, salt, and black pepper. Cook until the turkey is browned and cooked through, about 7-10 minutes. Break it up with a spoon as it cooks.
3. **Prepare Avocado**: In a small bowl, combine the diced avocado with lime juice. Gently mix to coat the avocado and prevent browning.
4. **Assemble the Wraps**: Take a lettuce leaf and spoon some of the turkey mixture into the center. Top with a few pieces of the lime-dressed avocado.

5. **Garnish**: If desired, sprinkle with fresh cilantro and serve with lime wedges on the side.

Cooking and Prep Time

- **Prep Time**: 10 minutes
- **Cook Time**: 15 minutes
- **Total Time**: 25 minutes
- **Servings**: 4

Nutrition Information (per serving)

- **Calories**: Approximately 250 kcal
- **Total Fat**: 14 g
- **Saturated Fat**: 2 g
- **Cholesterol**: 70 mg
- **Sodium**: 600 mg
- **Total Carbohydrates**: 10 g
- **Dietary Fiber**: 5 g
- **Sugars**: 1 g
- **Protein**: 25 g

6.2.7 Stuffed Bell Peppers

Ingredients

- **Bell Peppers**: 4-6 large bell peppers (any color)
- **Ground Meat**: 1 lb (lean ground beef, turkey, or Italian sausage)
- **Rice**: 1 cup uncooked white or brown rice
- **Onion**: 1 medium yellow onion, finely chopped
- **Garlic**: 3 cloves, minced
- **Tomato Sauce**: 1 (15-ounce) can or 1 cup marinara sauce
- **Broth**: 1 cup chicken or vegetable broth
- **Seasonings**:
    - 1 teaspoon Italian seasoning
    - 1 teaspoon salt
    - 1/2 teaspoon black pepper
    - 1 tablespoon Worcestershire sauce (optional)

- **Cheese**: 3/4 cup shredded cheese (cheddar or mozzarella) for topping
- **Olive Oil**: 1 tablespoon for sautéing

Directions

1. **Preheat the Oven**: Preheat your oven to 350°F (175°C).
2. **Prepare the Peppers**: Wash the bell peppers and cut the tops off. Remove the seeds and membranes. If needed, trim the bottoms slightly to help them stand upright.
3. **Par-Cook the Peppers**: Place the bell peppers in a baking dish and add a little water to the bottom. Cover with foil and bake for about 20 minutes to soften them.
4. **Cook the Filling**:
    - In a large skillet, heat olive oil over medium heat. Add the chopped onion and garlic, sautéing until the onion is translucent.

- ○ Add the ground meat and cook until browned. Drain excess fat if
    necessary.
  - ○ Stir in the rice, tomato sauce, broth, Worcestershire sauce, Italian
    seasoning, salt, and pepper. Bring to a boil, then reduce heat and simmer
    for about 20 minutes, or until the rice is tender.

5. **Stuff the Peppers**: Remove the peppers from the oven and fill each one with the meat and rice mixture. Pack the filling tightly.
6. **Bake**: Cover the stuffed peppers with foil and bake for an additional 25 minutes. Remove the foil, sprinkle cheese on top, and bake for another 10 minutes, or until the cheese is melted and bubbly.
7. **Serve**: Let the peppers cool slightly before serving. Enjoy!

Cooking and Prep Time

- **Prep Time**: 15-20 minutes
- **Cook Time**: 50-60 minutes
- **Total Time**: 1 hour 15 minutes
- **Servings**: 4-6

Nutrition Information (per stuffed pepper)

- **Calories**: Approximately 350 kcal
- **Total Fat**: 15 g
- **Saturated Fat**: 6 g
- **Cholesterol**: 70 mg
- **Sodium**: 600 mg
- **Total Carbohydrates**: 40 g
- **Dietary Fiber**: 5 g
- **Sugars**: 5 g
- **Protein**: 20 g

6.2.8 Asian Noodle Salad

Ingredients

- **Noodles**:
  - 8 ounces rice vermicelli noodles (or substitute with soba, egg noodles, or soy noodles)

- **Vegetables**:
  - 1 English cucumber, thinly sliced
  - 1 large carrot, shredded or thinly sliced
  - 2 cups green cabbage, shredded
  - 4 green onions (spring onions), sliced
  - 1 cup bean sprouts (optional)
  - 1/4 cup fresh cilantro, chopped (or substitute with parsley)

- **Dressing**:
  - 1/4 cup soy sauce (or Tamari for gluten-free)
  - 2 tablespoons sesame oil
  - 2 tablespoons lime juice (or rice vinegar)
  - 1 tablespoon honey or maple syrup
  - 1 clove garlic, minced
  - 1 teaspoon fresh ginger, grated (or 1/4 teaspoon ground ginger)
  - Red pepper flakes or fresh chili, to taste (optional)

- **Toppings**:
  - 1/4 cup chopped peanuts or sesame seeds (optional)

Directions

1. **Prepare the Noodles**: Cook the rice vermicelli noodles according to package instructions (usually soaking in hot water for about 5 minutes). Drain and rinse under cold water to stop the cooking process. Set aside.
2. **Make the Dressing**: In a small bowl, whisk together the soy sauce, sesame oil, lime juice, honey, minced garlic, grated ginger, and red pepper flakes until well combined.
3. **Combine the Salad**: In a large bowl, combine the cooked noodles, cucumber, carrot, cabbage, green onions, and bean sprouts. Pour the dressing over the salad and toss gently to combine.
4. **Add Herbs and Serve**: Fold in the chopped cilantro. If desired, top with chopped peanuts or sesame seeds for added crunch. Serve immediately or refrigerate for 30 minutes to allow the flavors to meld.

Cooking and Prep Time

- **Prep Time**: 15 minutes
- **Cook Time**: 5 minutes (for noodles)
- **Total Time**: 20 minutes
- **Servings**: 4-6

Nutrition Information (per serving)

- **Calories**: Approximately 200 kcal
- **Total Fat**: 10 g
- **Saturated Fat**: 1.5 g
- **Cholesterol**: 0 mg
- **Sodium**: 800 mg
- **Total Carbohydrates**: 25 g
- **Dietary Fiber**: 3 g
- **Sugars**: 5 g
- **Protein**: 5 g

6.2.9 Cauliflower Rice Bowl

Ingredients

- 2 cups cauliflower rice (from 1 small head of cauliflower)
- 2 ¾ cups cooked bulgur (about 1 cup dry)
- 2 cups vegetable broth
- 4 cups Romaine lettuce, chopped (or greens of choice)
- 1 cup celery, chopped
- ½ cup red onion, diced
- 1 (15-ounce) can Northern white beans, rinsed and drained
- 1 cup grape tomatoes, halved
- 1 cup English cucumber, cut into bite-sized pieces (about ½ cucumber)
- ½ cup tofu feta cheese (optional)
- Sunflower sprouts or microgreens for garnish (optional)

For the Lemon Tahini Dressing:

- ¼ cup tahini
- 3 tablespoons lemon juice
- ½ cup water
- 2 tablespoons apple cider vinegar
- 2 teaspoons Dijon mustard
- 2 teaspoons maple syrup
- ½ teaspoon sea salt
- ½ teaspoon black pepper

Directions

1. Make the cauliflower rice by pulsing cauliflower florets in a food processor until they resemble rice grains. Alternatively, grate the cauliflower using a box grater.
2. In a sauccpan, bring the vegetable broth to a boil. Add the dry bulgur, reduce the heat to low, cover, and simmer for about 12-15 minutes until the bulgur is tender. Fluff with a fork and set aside.

3. In a small bowl, whisk together all the ingredients for the lemon tahini dressing until smooth. Adjust the consistency with more water if needed.

4. In a large bowl, combine the cauliflower rice, cooked bulgur, chopped Romaine lettuce, celery, red onion, white beans, grape tomatoes, and cucumber. Toss gently to mix.

5. Drizzle the lemon tahini dressing over the salad and toss to combine. Top with tofu feta cheese and garnish with sunflower sprouts or microgreens if desired.

6. Serve immediately or refrigerate for up to 2 days. The flavors will meld beautifully if allowed to sit for a while.

Cooking and Prep Time

- Prep Time: 15 minutes
- Cook Time: 15 minutes
- Total Time: 30 minutes
- Servings: 4-6

Nutrition Information (per serving)

- Calories: Approximately 350 kcal
- Total Fat: 15 g
- Saturated Fat: 2 g
- Cholesterol: 0 mg
- Sodium: 400 mg
- Total Carbohydrates: 45 g
- Dietary Fiber: 10 g
- Sugars: 5 g
- Protein: 12 g

6.2.10 Chicken and Spinach Soup

Ingredients

- 1 lb boneless, skinless chicken breasts, cut into bite-sized pieces
- 1 tbsp olive oil
- 1 onion, diced
- 3 cloves garlic, minced
- 6 cups chicken broth
- 1 cup uncooked orzo pasta
- 4 cups fresh spinach, chopped
- 1 tsp dried thyme
- Salt and pepper to taste
- Grated Parmesan cheese for serving (optional)

Directions

1. **In a large pot**, heat the olive oil over medium heat. Add the diced onion and sauté for 3-4 minutes until translucent.
2. **Add the minced garlic** and cook for an additional minute until fragrant.
3. **Add the chicken pieces** to the pot and cook for 5-6 minutes, stirring occasionally, until the chicken is no longer pink.
4. **Pour in the chicken broth** and stir in the uncooked orzo pasta. Bring the soup to a boil.
5. **Once boiling, reduce heat** to medium-low and let the soup simmer for 8-10 minutes, or until the orzo is tender.
6. **Stir in the chopped spinach** and dried thyme. Cook for an additional 2-3 minutes until the spinach is wilted.
7. **Season with salt and pepper** to taste.
8. **Serve hot**, garnished with grated Parmesan cheese if desired.

Cooking and Prep Time

- **Prep Time**: 10 minutes
- **Cook Time**: 20 minutes
- **Total Time**: 30 minutes
- **Servings**: 4-6

Nutrition Information (per serving)

- **Calories**: Approximately 250 kcal
- **Total Fat**: 5 g
- **Saturated Fat**: 1 g
- **Cholesterol**: 65 mg
- **Sodium**: 800 mg
- **Total Carbohydrates**: 25 g
- **Dietary Fiber**: 2 g
- **Sugars**: 3 g
- **Protein**: 25 g

6.2.11 Avocado and Chickpea Salad

Ingredients

- 2 (15-ounce) cans chickpeas, drained and rinsed
- 2 ripe avocados, diced
- 1 cucumber, diced
- 1 pint cherry tomatoes, halved
- 1/2 red onion, thinly sliced
- 1/4 cup chopped fresh cilantro or parsley
- 2 tablespoons olive oil
- 2 tablespoons lemon juice
- 1 garlic clove, minced
- 1/2 teaspoon ground cumin
- 1/4 teaspoon cayenne pepper (optional)
- Salt and pepper to taste

Instructions

1. In a large bowl, combine the drained and rinsed chickpeas, diced avocado, cucumber, cherry tomatoes, red onion, and chopped cilantro or parsley.
2. In a small bowl, whisk together the olive oil, lemon juice, minced garlic, cumin, and cayenne pepper (if using). Season with salt and pepper to taste.
3. Pour the dressing over the chickpea and avocado mixture and gently toss to combine, being careful not to mash the avocado too much.
4. Serve immediately or refrigerate until ready to serve. The salad will keep well for up to 2 days in the refrigerator.

Cooking and Prep Time

- **Prep Time**: 15 minutes
- **Total Time**: 15 minutes
- **Servings**: 4-6

Nutrition Information (per serving)

- **Calories**: Approximately 300 kcal
- **Total Fat**: 15 g
- **Saturated Fat**: 2 g
- **Cholesterol**: 0 mg
- **Sodium**: 400 mg
- **Total Carbohydrates**: 35 g
- **Dietary Fiber**: 10 g
- **Sugars**: 5 g
- **Protein**: 10 g

6.2.12 Tuna Salad Stuffed Tomatoes

Ingredients

- 1 (5-ounce) can tuna packed in water, drained
- 2 tablespoons light mayonnaise
- 1½ tablespoons sweet pickle relish
- ½ stalk celery, diced
- ⅛ teaspoon celery salt
- ⅛ teaspoon ground black pepper
- 2 large ripe tomatoes
- ⅛ teaspoon kosher salt (for seasoning the tomatoes)
- Optional: minced parsley for garnish

Directions

1. **Prepare the Tuna Salad**: In a bowl, break up the drained tuna with a fork. Add the light mayonnaise, pickle relish, diced celery, celery salt, and black pepper. Mix until well combined. Taste and adjust the seasoning if necessary.
2. **Prepare the Tomatoes**: Cut the tops off the large tomatoes and scoop out the insides using a small spoon, leaving a thin layer of flesh next to the skin. Be careful not to break the tomatoes. Sprinkle a little kosher salt inside each hollowed-out tomato to enhance the flavor.
3. **Stuff the Tomatoes**: Use a small spoon to fill each tomato with the tuna salad mixture. Press down gently to ensure they're filled well.
4. **Garnish and Serve**: If desired, garnish with minced parsley. Serve immediately or refrigerate until ready to eat.

Cooking and Prep Time

- **Prep Time**: 10 minutes
- **Total Time**: 10 minutes
- **Servings**: 2

Nutrition Information (per stuffed tomato)

- **Calories**: Approximately 135 kcal
- **Total Fat**: 2.5 g
- **Saturated Fat**: 0.6 g
- **Cholesterol**: 29.8 mg
- **Sodium**: 522.5 mg
- **Total Carbohydrates**: 10.5 g
- **Dietary Fiber**: 2.2 g
- **Sugars**: 7.6 g
- **Protein**: 18.2 g

6.2.13 Zucchini Noodles with Pesto

Ingredients

- **For the Zucchini Noodles**:
    - 4 medium zucchinis, spiralized
    - 1 tablespoon olive oil
    - Salt and pepper to taste

- **For the Pesto**:
    - 2 cups fresh basil leaves
    - 1/2 cup grated Parmesan cheese
    - 1/3 cup pine nuts (or walnuts)
    - 2 garlic cloves
    - 1/2 cup olive oil
    - Salt and pepper to taste
    - Juice of 1 lemon (optional)

Directions

1. **Make the Pesto**:
    - In a food processor, combine the basil leaves, Parmesan cheese, pine nuts, and garlic cloves. Pulse until finely chopped.
    - With the processor running, slowly drizzle in the olive oil until the mixture is smooth. Season with salt and pepper to taste. If desired, add lemon juice for brightness.

2. **Prepare the Zucchini Noodles**:
    - Heat a large skillet over medium heat and add the olive oil.

- o Add the spiralized zucchini noodles to the skillet. Sauté for about 3-5 minutes, stirring occasionally, until the noodles are tender but still have a slight crunch. Season with salt and pepper.

3. **Combine**:
   - o Remove the skillet from heat and add the pesto to the zucchini noodles. Toss gently to combine, ensuring the noodles are evenly coated with the pesto.

4. **Serve**:
   - o Plate the zucchini noodles and garnish with additional Parmesan cheese and fresh basil if desired. Serve immediately.

Cooking and Prep Time

- **Prep Time**: 10 minutes
- **Cook Time**: 5 minutes
- **Total Time**: 15 minutes
- **Servings**: 4

Nutrition Information (per serving)

- **Calories**: Approximately 250 kcal
- **Total Fat**: 20 g
- **Saturated Fat**: 4 g
- **Cholesterol**: 10 mg
- **Sodium**: 200 mg
- **Total Carbohydrates**: 10 g
- **Dietary Fiber**: 3 g
- **Sugars**: 4 g
- **Protein**: 6 g

6.2.14 Spicy Black Bean and Corn Salad

Ingredients

- **For the Salad**:
    - 1 (15-ounce) can black beans, drained and rinsed
    - 1 cup corn (fresh, canned, or frozen)
    - 1 red bell pepper, diced
    - 1 small red onion, diced
    - 1 cup cherry tomatoes, halved
    - 1 avocado, diced
    - 1/4 cup fresh cilantro, chopped
    - 1 jalapeño, seeded and minced (optional, for extra heat)

- **For the Dressing**:
    - 3 tablespoons olive oil
    - 2 tablespoons lime juice (freshly squeezed)
    - 1 teaspoon cumin
    - 1 teaspoon chili powder
    - Salt and pepper to taste

Directions

1. **Prepare the Salad Ingredients**: In a large bowl, combine the black beans, corn, diced red bell pepper, diced red onion, halved cherry tomatoes, diced avocado, chopped cilantro, and minced jalapeño (if using).
2. **Make the Dressing**: In a small bowl, whisk together the olive oil, lime juice, cumin, chili powder, salt, and pepper until well combined.
3. **Combine**: Pour the dressing over the salad mixture and gently toss to coat all the ingredients evenly.

4. **Serve**: Let the salad sit for about 10 minutes to allow the flavors to meld. Serve chilled or at room temperature.

Cooking and Prep Time

- **Prep Time**: 15 minutes
- **Total Time**: 15 minutes
- **Servings**: 4-6

Nutrition Information (per serving)

- **Calories**: Approximately 180 kcal
- **Total Fat**: 9 g
- **Saturated Fat**: 1 g
- **Cholesterol**: 0 mg
- **Sodium**: 250 mg
- **Total Carbohydrates**: 22 g
- **Dietary Fiber**: 7 g
- **Sugars**: 3 g
- **Protein**: 6 g

6.2.15 Butternut Squash and Lentil Curry

Ingredients

- 1 medium butternut squash (about 2 lbs), peeled and diced
- 1 cup red lentils, rinsed
- 1 tablespoon olive oil
- 1 onion, chopped
- 3 garlic cloves, minced
- 1 tablespoon fresh ginger, grated
- 1 teaspoon ground cumin
- 1 teaspoon ground coriander
- 1 teaspoon turmeric
- 1/2 teaspoon cayenne pepper (adjust to taste)
- 1 (14-ounce) can coconut milk
- 4 cups vegetable broth
- Salt and pepper to taste
- Fresh cilantro for garnish (optional)
- Lime wedges for serving (optional)

Directions

1. **Sauté the Aromatics**: In a large pot, heat the olive oil over medium heat. Add the chopped onion and sauté for about 5 minutes until softened. Stir in the minced garlic and grated ginger, cooking for an additional 1-2 minutes until fragrant.
2. **Add Spices**: Sprinkle in the ground cumin, coriander, turmeric, and cayenne pepper. Stir well to coat the onion mixture with the spices and cook for another minute.
3. **Combine Ingredients**: Add the diced butternut squash, rinsed lentils, coconut milk, and vegetable broth to the pot. Stir to combine all ingredients.

4. **Simmer**: Bring the mixture to a boil, then reduce the heat to low. Cover and let it simmer for about 25-30 minutes, or until the squash is tender and the lentils are cooked through. Stir occasionally and add more broth or water if needed to reach your desired consistency.

5. **Season and Serve**: Taste the curry and season with salt and pepper. Serve hot, garnished with fresh cilantro and lime wedges if desired.

Cooking and Prep Time

- **Prep Time**: 15 minutes
- **Cook Time**: 30 minutes
- **Total Time**: 45 minutes
- **Servings**: 4-6

Nutrition Information (per serving)

- **Calories**: Approximately 300 kcal
- **Total Fat**: 10 g
- **Saturated Fat**: 5 g
- **Cholesterol**: 0 mg
- **Sodium**: 400 mg
- **Total Carbohydrates**: 45 g
- **Dietary Fiber**: 12 g
- **Sugars**: 5 g
- **Protein**: 12 g

6.3 Dinner

6.3.1 Grilled Salmon with Asparagus

Ingredients

- **4** salmon fillets (about 6 ounces each)
- **1 lb** asparagus spears, trimmed
- **2 tbsp** olive oil
- **1 tsp** lemon zest
- **2 tbsp** lemon juice
- **1 tsp** dried dill
- **1/2 tsp** salt
- **1/4 tsp** black pepper

Directions

1. **Preheat** your grill to medium-high heat.
2. **In a large bowl**, combine the trimmed asparagus spears, 1 tbsp olive oil, 1/4 tsp salt, and 1/8 tsp black pepper. Toss to coat the asparagus evenly.
3. **Place the asparagus** on a grill basket or directly on the grill grates. Grill for 5-7 minutes, turning occasionally, until tender and slightly charred.
4. **In a small bowl**, mix together the remaining 1 tbsp olive oil, lemon zest, lemon juice, dried dill, 1/4 tsp salt, and 1/8 tsp black pepper. Set aside.
5. **Season the salmon fillets** with the remaining 1/4 tsp salt and 1/8 tsp black pepper.
6. **Place the salmon fillets**, skin-side down, on the grill grates. Grill for 4-6 minutes per side, or until the salmon flakes easily with a fork and reaches an internal temperature of 145°F.
7. **Drizzle the lemon-dill mixture** over the grilled salmon and asparagus.
8. **Serve immediately**, garnished with additional lemon wedges if desired.

Cooking and Prep Time

- **Prep Time**: 10 minutes
- **Cook Time**: 15 minutes
- **Total Time**: 25 minutes
- **Servings**: 4

Nutrition Information (per serving)

- **Calories**: Approximately 300 kcal
- **Total Fat**: 16 g
- **Saturated Fat**: 3 g
- **Cholesterol**: 90 mg
- **Sodium**: 500 mg
- **Total Carbohydrates**: 6 g
- **Dietary Fiber**: 3 g
- **Sugars**: 2 g
- **Protein**: 35 g

6.3.2 Chicken Stir-Fry

Ingredients

- **For the Stir-Fry**:
  - 1 lb boneless, skinless chicken breasts, thinly sliced
  - 2 tablespoons vegetable oil (divided)
  - 1 bell pepper (red or green), sliced
  - 1 cup broccoli florets
  - 1 cup snap peas (or snow peas)
  - 1 carrot, thinly sliced
  - 3 cloves garlic, minced
  - 1 tablespoon fresh ginger, minced
  - 3 green onions, chopped

- **For the Sauce**:
  - 1/4 cup soy sauce (or tamari for gluten-free)
  - 2 tablespoons oyster sauce (or hoisin sauce)
  - 1 tablespoon cornstarch
  - 1 tablespoon honey or brown sugar
  - 1 tablespoon rice vinegar or apple cider vinegar
  - 1 teaspoon sesame oil (optional)
  - Red pepper flakes (optional, to taste)

Directions

1. **Prepare the Sauce**: In a small bowl, whisk together the soy sauce, oyster sauce, cornstarch, honey, rice vinegar, and sesame oil. Set aside.
2. **Cook the Chicken**: Heat 1 tablespoon of vegetable oil in a large skillet or wok over medium-high heat. Add the sliced chicken and cook for 5-7 minutes, or until

the chicken is cooked through and no longer pink. Remove the chicken from the skillet and set aside.

3. **Stir-Fry the Vegetables**: In the same skillet, add the remaining tablespoon of vegetable oil. Add the sliced bell pepper, broccoli, snap peas, and carrot. Stir-fry for about 3-5 minutes until the vegetables are tender-crisp.

4. **Add Garlic and Ginger**: Add the minced garlic and ginger to the skillet, stirring for about 30 seconds until fragrant.

5. **Combine Chicken and Sauce**: Return the cooked chicken to the skillet. Pour the prepared sauce over the chicken and vegetables. Stir well to combine and cook for an additional 2-3 minutes until the sauce thickens.

6. **Garnish and Serve**: Remove from heat and stir in the chopped green onions. Serve hot over rice or noodles, and garnish with red pepper flakes if desired.

Cooking and Prep Time

- **Prep Time**: 15 minutes
- **Cook Time**: 15 minutes
- **Total Time**: 30 minutes
- **Servings**: 4

Nutrition Information (per serving)

- **Calories**: Approximately 300 kcal
- **Total Fat**: 10 g
- **Saturated Fat**: 1.5 g
- **Cholesterol**: 70 mg
- **Sodium**: 800 mg
- **Total Carbohydrates**: 25 g
- **Dietary Fiber**: 3 g
- **Sugars**: 5 g
- **Protein**: 30 g

6.3.3 Beef and Broccoli

Ingredients

- 1 lb flank steak or sirloin, thinly sliced against the grain
- 1 head broccoli, cut into florets (about 4 cups)
- 2 tablespoons vegetable oil, divided
- 3 cloves garlic, minced
- 1 tablespoon grated fresh ginger
- 1/4 cup low-sodium soy sauce
- 2 tablespoons brown sugar
- 1 tablespoon rice vinegar
- 1 teaspoon sesame oil
- 1/4 teaspoon red pepper flakes (optional)
- 2 teaspoons cornstarch
- 2 tablespoons water
- Salt and pepper to taste
- Sesame seeds for garnish (optional)

Directions

1. **In a bowl**, whisk together 1 tablespoon soy sauce, 1 tablespoon brown sugar, 1 teaspoon sesame oil, and 1 teaspoon cornstarch. Add the sliced beef and toss to coat. Cover and refrigerate for 30 minutes to 1 hour.
2. **In a small bowl**, whisk together the remaining 3 tablespoons soy sauce, 1 tablespoon brown sugar, rice vinegar, and red pepper flakes (if using). Set aside.
3. **In a large skillet or wok**, heat 1 tablespoon vegetable oil over high heat. Add the marinated beef in a single layer and cook undisturbed for 1 minute to sear. Flip and cook for another minute. Transfer beef to a plate.
4. **Add the remaining 1 tablespoon vegetable oil to the skillet**. Add the broccoli florets and stir-fry for 2-3 minutes until crisp-tender.
5. **Add the garlic and ginger** and cook for 1 minute until fragrant.

6. **Return the beef and any accumulated juices** to the skillet. Pour in the soy sauce mixture and bring to a simmer.

7. **In a small bowl**, whisk together the remaining 1 teaspoon cornstarch and 2 tablespoons water. Pour into the skillet and cook for 1-2 minutes until the sauce thickens slightly.

8. **Remove from heat** and season with salt and pepper to taste.

9. **Serve immediately** over steamed rice, garnished with sesame seeds if desired.

Cooking and Prep Time

- **Prep Time**: 15 minutes (plus marinating time)
- **Cook Time**: 10 minutes
- **Total Time**: 25 minutes (plus marinating time)
- **Servings**: 4

Nutrition Information (per serving)

- **Calories**: Approximately 300 kcal
- **Total Fat**: 12 g
- **Saturated Fat**: 3 g
- **Cholesterol**: 60 mg
- **Sodium**: 700 mg
- **Total Carbohydrates**: 18 g
- **Dietary Fiber**: 3 g
- **Sugars**: 8 g
- **Protein**: 30 g

6.3.4 Stuffed Acorn Squash

Ingredients

- **For the Squash**:
    - 2 medium acorn squashes, halved and seeds removed
    - 2 tablespoons olive oil
    - Salt and pepper to taste

- **For the Filling**:
    - 1 cup cooked quinoa (or rice)
    - 1 cup cooked black beans (canned, drained, and rinsed)
    - 1 cup corn (fresh, canned, or frozen)
    - 1 bell pepper, diced
    - 1 small red onion, diced
    - 2 cloves garlic, minced
    - 1 teaspoon ground cumin
    - 1 teaspoon chili powder
    - 1/2 teaspoon smoked paprika
    - 1/4 cup fresh cilantro, chopped (optional)
    - 1/2 cup shredded cheese (cheddar or pepper jack, optional)

Directions

1. **Prepare the Squash**: Preheat the oven to 400°F (200°C). Cut the acorn squashes in half and scoop out the seeds. Brush the cut sides with olive oil and sprinkle with salt and pepper. Place the squash halves cut-side down on a baking sheet and roast for 25-30 minutes until tender.
2. **Make the Filling**: In a large skillet, heat a tablespoon of olive oil over medium heat. Add the diced red onion and bell pepper, cooking until softened, about 5

minutes. Add the minced garlic, cumin, chili powder, and smoked paprika, cooking for an additional minute until fragrant.

3. **Combine Ingredients**: In a large bowl, combine the cooked quinoa, black beans, corn, sautéed vegetables, and chopped cilantro (if using). Mix well and adjust seasoning with salt and pepper to taste.

4. **Stuff the Squash**: Remove the roasted acorn squash from the oven and carefully flip them cut-side up. Spoon the filling into each squash half, pressing down gently to pack it in. If desired, sprinkle shredded cheese on top.

5. **Bake Again**: Return the stuffed squashes to the oven and bake for an additional 10-15 minutes until heated through and the cheese is melted.

6. **Serve**: Remove from the oven and let cool slightly before serving. Enjoy warm!

Cooking and Prep Time

- **Prep Time**: 15 minutes
- **Cook Time**: 45 minutes
- **Total Time**: 1 hour
- **Servings**: 4

Nutrition Information (per stuffed squash half)

- **Calories**: Approximately 300 kcal
- **Total Fat**: 10 g
- **Saturated Fat**: 3 g
- **Cholesterol**: 15 mg (if cheese is used)
- **Sodium**: 400 mg
- **Total Carbohydrates**: 45 g
- **Dietary Fiber**: 10 g
- **Sugars**: 4 g
- **Protein**: 10 g

6.3.5 Lemon Herb Chicken Thighs

Ingredients

- **8** bone-in, skin-on chicken thighs
- **2 tbsp** olive oil
- **1 tbsp** lemon zest
- **2 tbsp** lemon juice
- **1 tsp** dried oregano
- **1 tsp** dried basil
- **1 tsp** dried thyme
- **1 tsp** salt
- **1/2 tsp** black pepper
- **2 cloves** garlic, minced
- **1/4 cup** chopped fresh parsley

Directions

1. **Preheat** your oven to 400°F (200°C).
2. **In a large bowl**, combine the olive oil, lemon zest, lemon juice, oregano, basil, thyme, salt, and black pepper. Add the chicken thighs and toss to coat evenly.
3. **Arrange** the chicken thighs skin-side up on a large baking sheet lined with parchment paper or a silicone baking mat.
4. **Bake** for 30-35 minutes, or until the chicken is cooked through and the skin is crispy. The internal temperature should reach 165°F (75°C).
5. **In the last 5 minutes** of cooking, sprinkle the minced garlic over the chicken.
6. **Remove** the chicken from the oven and let it rest for 5 minutes.
7. **Garnish** with chopped fresh parsley before serving.

Cooking and Prep Time

- **Prep Time**: 10 minutes
- **Cook Time**: 35 minutes
- **Total Time**: 45 minutes

- **Servings**: 4

Nutrition Information (per serving)

- **Calories**: Approximately 350 kcal
- **Total Fat**: 25 g
- **Saturated Fat**: 7 g
- **Cholesterol**: 165 mg
- **Sodium**: 650 mg
- **Total Carbohydrates**: 2 g
- **Dietary Fiber**: 0 g
- **Sugars**: 0 g
- **Protein**: 35 g

6.3.6 Eggplant Parmesan

Ingredients

- **For the Eggplant**:
    - 2 medium eggplants, sliced into 1/4-inch rounds
    - 1 teaspoon salt
    - 1 cup all-purpose flour
    - 2 large eggs, beaten
    - 2 cups breadcrumbs (preferably Italian-style)
    - 1/2 cup grated Parmesan cheese
    - 1/2 teaspoon black pepper
    - Olive oil for frying

- **For the Assembly**:
    - 4 cups marinara sauce (store-bought or homemade)
    - 2 cups shredded mozzarella cheese
    - Fresh basil leaves for garnish (optional)

Directions

1. **Prepare the Eggplant**:
    - Sprinkle the eggplant slices with salt and let them sit in a colander for about 30 minutes. This helps draw out excess moisture and bitterness. Rinse and pat dry with paper towels.

2. **Set Up Breading Station**:
    - In three separate shallow dishes, place the flour, beaten eggs, and a mixture of breadcrumbs, grated Parmesan cheese, and black pepper.

3. **Bread the Eggplant**:
   - Dip each eggplant slice into the flour, shaking off the excess, then into the beaten eggs, and finally coat with the breadcrumb mixture. Press gently to adhere.

4. **Fry the Eggplant**:
   - In a large skillet, heat olive oil over medium heat. Fry the breaded eggplant slices in batches, about 3-4 minutes per side, until golden brown. Remove and place on paper towels to drain excess oil.

5. **Assemble the Dish**:
   - Preheat your oven to 375°F (190°C). In a baking dish, spread a layer of marinara sauce on the bottom. Layer half of the fried eggplant slices, followed by half of the remaining marinara sauce, and half of the mozzarella cheese. Repeat the layers with the remaining eggplant, marinara sauce, and mozzarella cheese on top.

6. **Bake**:
   - Cover the baking dish with foil and bake for 25 minutes. Remove the foil and bake for an additional 15 minutes, or until the cheese is bubbly and golden.

7. **Garnish and Serve**:
   - Let the dish cool for a few minutes before slicing. Garnish with fresh basil leaves if desired, and serve hot.

Cooking and Prep Time

- **Prep Time**: 30 minutes (plus 30 minutes for salting the eggplant)
- **Cook Time**: 40 minutes
- **Total Time**: 1 hour 40 minutes

- **Servings**: 6

Nutrition Information (per serving)

- **Calories**: Approximately 350 kcal
- **Total Fat**: 20 g
- **Saturated Fat**: 8 g
- **Cholesterol**: 150 mg
- **Sodium**: 800 mg
- **Total Carbohydrates**: 30 g
- **Dietary Fiber**: 6 g
- **Sugars**: 6 g
- **Protein**: 15 g

6.3.7 Shrimp and Vegetable Skewers

Ingredients

- **For the Skewers**:
    - 1 lb large shrimp, peeled and deveined
    - 1 red bell pepper, cut into chunks
    - 1 zucchini, sliced into rounds
    - 1 yellow squash, sliced into rounds
    - 1 red onion, cut into chunks
    - 2 tablespoons olive oil
    - 2 tablespoons lemon juice
    - 3 cloves garlic, minced
    - 1 teaspoon dried oregano
    - 1 teaspoon paprika
    - Salt and pepper to taste
    - Skewers (wooden or metal)

Directions

1. **Prepare the Skewers**: If using wooden skewers, soak them in water for at least 30 minutes to prevent burning on the grill.
2. **Make the Marinade**: In a large bowl, whisk together the olive oil, lemon juice, minced garlic, dried oregano, paprika, salt, and pepper.
3. **Marinate the Shrimp and Vegetables**: Add the shrimp, bell pepper, zucchini, yellow squash, and red onion to the bowl. Toss to coat everything evenly with the marinade. Let it marinate for about 15-30 minutes.
4. **Assemble the Skewers**: Thread the marinated shrimp and vegetables onto the skewers, alternating between shrimp and vegetables.
5. **Preheat the Grill**: Heat the grill to medium-high heat.

6. **Grill the Skewers**: Place the skewers on the grill and cook for about 2-3 minutes per side, or until the shrimp are pink and opaque and the vegetables are tender.

7. **Serve**: Remove the skewers from the grill and serve immediately, garnished with fresh herbs or lemon wedges if desired.

Cooking and Prep Time

- **Prep Time**: 15 minutes (plus marinating time)
- **Cook Time**: 10 minutes
- **Total Time**: 25-35 minutes
- **Servings**: 4

Nutrition Information (per serving)

- **Calories**: Approximately 220 kcal
- **Total Fat**: 10 g
- **Saturated Fat**: 1 g
- **Cholesterol**: 200 mg
- **Sodium**: 300 mg
- **Total Carbohydrates**: 10 g
- **Dietary Fiber**: 2 g
- **Sugars**: 3 g
- **Protein**: 25 g

6.3.8 Turkey Meatballs with Zucchini Noodles

Ingredients

- **For the Turkey Meatballs**:
    - 1 lb ground turkey
    - 1/2 cup breadcrumbs (or almond flour for a low-carb option)
    - 1/4 cup grated Parmesan cheese
    - 1 large egg
    - 2 cloves garlic, minced
    - 1 tablespoon fresh parsley, chopped (or 1 teaspoon dried)
    - 1 teaspoon Italian seasoning
    - Salt and pepper to taste

- **For the Zucchini Noodles**:
    - 4 medium zucchinis, spiralized
    - 2 tablespoons olive oil
    - 2 cloves garlic, minced
    - Salt and pepper to taste
    - 1/4 cup marinara sauce (optional, for serving)
    - Fresh basil for garnish (optional)

Directions

1. **Preheat the Oven**: Preheat your oven to 400°F (200°C).
2. **Make the Meatballs**:
    - In a large bowl, combine the ground turkey, breadcrumbs, Parmesan cheese, egg, minced garlic, parsley, Italian seasoning, salt, and pepper. Mix until just combined.
    - Form the mixture into meatballs, about 1 to 1.5 inches in diameter, and place them on a baking sheet lined with parchment paper.

3. **Bake the Meatballs**: Bake the meatballs in the preheated oven for about 20-25 minutes, or until they are cooked through and reach an internal temperature of 165°F (75°C).

4. **Prepare the Zucchini Noodles**:
   - While the meatballs are baking, heat olive oil in a large skillet over medium heat. Add the minced garlic and sauté for about 30 seconds until fragrant.
   - Add the spiralized zucchini noodles to the skillet. Sauté for 3-5 minutes, or until the noodles are tender but still slightly firm. Season with salt and pepper to taste.

5. **Serve**:
   - Divide the zucchini noodles among plates, top with turkey meatballs, and drizzle with marinara sauce if desired. Garnish with fresh basil.

Cooking and Prep Time

- **Prep Time**: 15 minutes
- **Cook Time**: 25 minutes
- **Total Time**: 40 minutes
- **Servings**: 4

Nutrition Information (per serving)

- **Calories**: Approximately 300 kcal
- **Total Fat**: 15 g
- **Saturated Fat**: 4 g
- **Cholesterol**: 120 mg
- **Sodium**: 400 mg
- **Total Carbohydrates**: 15 g
- **Dietary Fiber**: 3 g
- **Sugars**: 4 g
- **Protein**: 30 g

6.3.9 Baked Cod with Spinach and Tomatoes

Ingredients

- 1 lb cod fillets, cut into 4 portions
- 2 tablespoons olive oil
- 1 pint cherry tomatoes, halved
- 4 cups fresh spinach
- 3 cloves garlic, minced
- 1 teaspoon dried oregano
- 1/2 teaspoon salt
- 1/4 teaspoon black pepper
- 1/4 cup white wine or chicken broth
- 2 tablespoons lemon juice
- 1/4 cup grated Parmesan cheese (optional)

Directions

1. **Preheat** your oven to 400°F (200°C).
2. **In a large oven-safe skillet or baking dish**, arrange the cod fillets in a single layer.
3. **In a bowl**, combine the halved cherry tomatoes, fresh spinach, minced garlic, dried oregano, salt, and black pepper. Toss to mix well.
4. **Spoon** the tomato-spinach mixture over and around the cod fillets.
5. **Pour** the white wine or chicken broth and lemon juice over the top.
6. **Bake** for 15-20 minutes, or until the cod is opaque and flakes easily with a fork and the tomatoes are softened.
7. **Remove** from the oven and sprinkle with grated Parmesan cheese, if desired.
8. **Serve** immediately, garnished with fresh herbs if desired.

Cooking and Prep Time

- **Prep Time**: 10 minutes

- **Cook Time**: 20 minutes
- **Total Time**: 30 minutes
- **Servings**: 4

Nutrition Information (per serving)

- **Calories**: Approximately 250 kcal
- **Total Fat**: 10 g
- **Saturated Fat**: 2 g
- **Cholesterol**: 70 mg
- **Sodium**: 500 mg
- **Total Carbohydrates**: 10 g
- **Dietary Fiber**: 3 g
- **Sugars**: 3 g
- **Protein**: 30 g

6.3.10 Spaghetti Squash with Marinara Sauce

Ingredients

- **For the Spaghetti Squash**:
    - 1 medium spaghetti squash
    - 2 tablespoons olive oil
    - Salt and pepper to taste

- **For the Marinara Sauce**:
    - 2 tablespoons olive oil
    - 1/2 medium onion, chopped
    - 3 cloves garlic, minced
    - 1 (28-ounce) can crushed tomatoes
    - 1 teaspoon dried oregano
    - 1 teaspoon dried basil
    - 1/2 teaspoon salt
    - 1/4 teaspoon black pepper
    - 1 tablespoon sugar (optional, to balance acidity)
    - Fresh basil for garnish (optional)

Directions

1. **Prepare the Spaghetti Squash**:
    - Preheat your oven to 400°F (200°C).
    - Cut the spaghetti squash in half lengthwise and scoop out the seeds. Drizzle the inside with olive oil and season with salt and pepper.
    - Place the squash cut-side down on a baking sheet lined with parchment paper. Roast for 30-40 minutes, or until the flesh is tender and easily shredded with a fork.

2. **Make the Marinara Sauce**:
   - While the squash is roasting, heat olive oil in a large saucepan over medium heat. Add the chopped onion and sauté until soft and translucent, about 5 minutes.
   - Add the minced garlic and cook for an additional minute until fragrant.
   - Stir in the crushed tomatoes, oregano, basil, salt, pepper, and sugar (if using). Bring to a simmer and let it cook for about 15-20 minutes, stirring occasionally.

3. **Combine and Serve**:
   - Once the spaghetti squash is done, use a fork to scrape the flesh into strands.
   - Serve the spaghetti squash topped with the marinara sauce. Garnish with fresh basil if desired.

Cooking and Prep Time

- **Prep Time**: 10 minutes
- **Cook Time**: 40 minutes
- **Total Time**: 50 minutes
- **Servings**: 4

Nutrition Information (per serving)

- **Calories**: Approximately 200 kcal
- **Total Fat**: 10 g
- **Saturated Fat**: 1.5 g
- **Cholesterol**: 0 mg
- **Sodium**: 400 mg
- **Total Carbohydrates**: 24 g
- **Dietary Fiber**: 6 g
- **Sugars**: 5 g
- **Protein**: 4 g

6.3.11 Chili with Beans

Ingredients

- **For the Chili**:
    - 1 lb ground beef (or turkey for a lighter option)
    - 1 medium onion, chopped
    - 2 cloves garlic, minced
    - 1 bell pepper, chopped (any color)
    - 1 (14.5-ounce) can diced tomatoes (with juices)
    - 1 (15-ounce) can kidney beans, drained and rinsed
    - 1 (15-ounce) can black beans, drained and rinsed
    - 2 tablespoons chili powder
    - 1 teaspoon ground cumin
    - 1 teaspoon smoked paprika
    - 1/2 teaspoon salt
    - 1/4 teaspoon black pepper
    - 1 cup beef broth (or vegetable broth)
    - Optional toppings: shredded cheese, sour cream, chopped green onions, or cilantro

Directions

1. **Cook the Meat**: In a large pot or Dutch oven, heat a tablespoon of oil over medium heat. Add the ground beef and cook until browned, breaking it apart with a spoon, about 5-7 minutes. Drain excess fat if necessary.
2. **Sauté Vegetables**: Add the chopped onion, minced garlic, and bell pepper to the pot. Cook for about 5 minutes, or until the vegetables are softened.
3. **Add Spices**: Stir in the chili powder, cumin, smoked paprika, salt, and black pepper. Cook for an additional minute until fragrant.

4. **Combine Ingredients**: Add the diced tomatoes (with juices), kidney beans, black beans, and beef broth to the pot. Stir to combine all ingredients.

5. **Simmer**: Bring the chili to a boil, then reduce the heat to low. Cover and let it simmer for 20-30 minutes, stirring occasionally. If the chili is too thick, add more broth or water to reach your desired consistency.

6. **Serve**: Taste and adjust seasoning if necessary. Serve hot, topped with your choice of shredded cheese, sour cream, chopped green onions, or cilantro.

Cooking and Prep Time

- **Prep Time**: 10 minutes
- **Cook Time**: 30 minutes
- **Total Time**: 40 minutes
- **Servings**: 4-6

Nutrition Information (per serving)

- **Calories**: Approximately 350 kcal
- **Total Fat**: 15 g
- **Saturated Fat**: 5 g
- **Cholesterol**: 70 mg
- **Sodium**: 600 mg
- **Total Carbohydrates**: 35 g
- **Dietary Fiber**: 10 g
- **Sugars**: 3 g
- **Protein**: 25 g

6.3.12 Thai Coconut Curry

Ingredients

- **For the Curry**:
    - 2 tablespoons coconut oil (or vegetable oil)
    - 1 batch of Thai red curry paste (or 2-3 tablespoons store-bought)
    - 1 lb protein of choice (chicken, shrimp, tofu, or beef), cut into bite-sized pieces
    - 1 can (14 oz) coconut milk
    - 1 cup vegetable or chicken broth
    - 2 cups mixed vegetables (such as bell peppers, broccoli, and carrots)
    - 3 tablespoons fish sauce (or soy sauce for a vegetarian option)
    - 1 tablespoon brown sugar (or palm sugar)
    - Juice of 1 lime
    - Fresh basil or cilantro for garnish

Directions

1. **Heat the Oil**: In a large pot or wok, heat the coconut oil over medium-high heat. Once hot, add the Thai red curry paste and sauté for about 1-2 minutes until fragrant.
2. **Add Protein**: Add your choice of protein (chicken, shrimp, tofu, or beef) to the pot. Cook for about 5-7 minutes until the protein is nearly cooked through.
3. **Incorporate Coconut Milk**: Pour in the coconut milk and broth, stirring to combine. Bring the mixture to a gentle simmer.
4. **Add Vegetables**: Add the mixed vegetables to the pot. Simmer for another 5-10 minutes, or until the vegetables are tender and the protein is fully cooked.
5. **Season**: Stir in the fish sauce, brown sugar, and lime juice. Taste and adjust seasoning as needed.

6. **Serve**: Remove from heat and serve hot, garnished with fresh basil or cilantro. Enjoy over steamed rice or noodles.

Cooking and Prep Time

- **Prep Time**: 10 minutes
- **Cook Time**: 20 minutes
- **Total Time**: 30 minutes
- **Servings**: 4

Nutrition Information (per serving)

- **Calories**: Approximately 350 kcal
- **Total Fat**: 22 g
- **Saturated Fat**: 14 g
- **Cholesterol**: Varies by protein choice
- **Sodium**: 800 mg
- **Total Carbohydrates**: 30 g
- **Dietary Fiber**: 4 g
- **Sugars**: 5 g
- **Protein**: 15 g (varies by protein choice)

6.3.13 Roasted Vegetable Medley

Ingredients

- **Vegetables**:
    - 2 cups broccoli florets
    - 2 cups cauliflower florets
    - 2 cups carrots, sliced
    - 1 red bell pepper, chopped
    - 1 yellow bell pepper, chopped
    - 1 zucchini, sliced
    - 1 red onion, cut into wedges

- **For Seasoning**:
    - 3 tablespoons olive oil
    - 2 teaspoons garlic powder
    - 1 teaspoon dried thyme
    - 1 teaspoon dried oregano
    - Salt and pepper to taste
    - Fresh parsley for garnish (optional)

Directions

1. **Preheat the Oven**: Preheat your oven to 425°F (220°C).
2. **Prepare the Vegetables**: In a large mixing bowl, combine all the chopped vegetables.
3. **Season the Vegetables**: Drizzle the olive oil over the vegetables. Sprinkle with garlic powder, thyme, oregano, salt, and pepper. Toss everything together until the vegetables are evenly coated.
4. **Roast the Vegetables**: Spread the seasoned vegetables in a single layer on a large baking sheet. Make sure they are not overcrowded to ensure even roasting.

5. **Bake**: Roast in the preheated oven for 25-30 minutes, or until the vegetables are tender and slightly caramelized, stirring halfway through for even cooking.

6. **Serve**: Remove from the oven and garnish with fresh parsley if desired. Serve warm as a side dish or over grains for a light main course.

Cooking and Prep Time

- **Prep Time**: 15 minutes
- **Cook Time**: 30 minutes
- **Total Time**: 45 minutes
- **Servings**: 4-6

Nutrition Information (per serving)

- **Calories**: Approximately 150 kcal
- **Total Fat**: 7 g
- **Saturated Fat**: 1 g
- **Cholesterol**: 0 mg
- **Sodium**: 200 mg
- **Total Carbohydrates**: 20 g
- **Dietary Fiber**: 6 g
- **Sugars**: 5 g
- **Protein**: 4 g

6.3.14 Grilled Portobello Mushrooms with Garlic

Ingredients

- **Mushrooms**: 4 large portobello mushrooms, stems and gills removed, wiped clean
- **Marinade**:
    - ¼ cup balsamic vinegar
    - 1 tablespoon extra virgin olive oil
    - 1 tablespoon low sodium soy sauce
    - 1 tablespoon chopped fresh rosemary (or ½ teaspoon dried)
    - 1 teaspoon garlic powder
    - ½ teaspoon black pepper
    - ⅛ teaspoon cayenne pepper (optional)

- **For grilling**: Canola or vegetable oil

Directions

1. **Prepare the Marinade**: In a shallow baking dish, whisk together the balsamic vinegar, olive oil, soy sauce, rosemary, garlic powder, black pepper, and cayenne. Adjust seasonings to taste.
2. **Marinate the Mushrooms**: Add the portobello mushrooms to the marinade, turning to coat. Let them marinate for 5 minutes on one side, then flip and marinate for an additional 5 minutes. For a more intense flavor, you can marinate them for up to 30 minutes.
3. **Preheat the Grill**: Heat a grill or large skillet over medium heat (about 350 to 400 degrees F). Brush the grill with oil to prevent sticking.
4. **Grill the Mushrooms**: Remove the mushrooms from the marinade, shaking off any excess. Grill for 3-4 minutes on each side, basting with the reserved marinade several times during cooking, until they are caramelized and deep golden brown.

5. **Serve**: Serve the grilled mushrooms as is or top them with an herby avocado sauce or your favorite toppings like cheese, spinach, and tomato.

Cooking and Prep Time

- **Prep Time**: 10 minutes
- **Marinating Time**: 10-30 minutes (optional)
- **Cook Time**: 10-15 minutes
- **Total Time**: Approximately 30-55 minutes

Serving

This recipe serves 4, with each serving consisting of one large portobello mushroom. They can be served as a main dish or sliced and used in salads, sandwiches, or as a side dish.

Nutritional Information (per serving)

- **Calories**: Approximately 96 kcal
- **Carbohydrates**: 9 g
- **Protein**: 3 g
- **Fat**: 8 g
- **Saturated Fat**: 1 g
- **Sodium**: 598 mg
- **Potassium**: 500 mg
- **Fiber**: 2 g
- **Sugar**: 6 g

6.3.15 Lamb Chops with Mint Yogurt Sauce

Ingredients

For the Lamb Chops:

- 6-8 lamb chops, about 1-inch thick
- 2 tablespoons olive oil
- Salt and freshly ground black pepper

For the Mint Yogurt Sauce:

- 2 cups loosely packed fresh mint leaves
- 1 cup Greek yogurt
- 2 garlic cloves, minced
- 1 tablespoon fresh lemon juice
- 1/2 teaspoon ground cumin
- 1/4 teaspoon cayenne pepper (optional)
- Salt and freshly ground black pepper to taste

Directions

1. **Make the Mint Yogurt Sauce:** In a food processor or blender, combine the mint leaves, yogurt, garlic, lemon juice, cumin, cayenne (if using), salt, and pepper. Blend until smooth and creamy. Transfer to a bowl and refrigerate until ready to serve.
2. **Cook the Lamb Chops:** Season the lamb chops generously with salt and pepper on both sides.
3. **In a large skillet, heat the olive oil over medium-high heat**. Working in batches if needed, add the lamb chops and cook for 3-4 minutes per side, until nicely browned. Adjust heat as needed to prevent burning.
4. Transfer the skillet to a preheated 400°F oven and roast for 5-8 minutes, depending on thickness, until chops reach desired doneness (125°F for medium-rare, 130-135°F for medium).
5. Remove the chops from the oven and let rest for 5 minutes before serving.

6. Serve the lamb chops warm, drizzled with a bit of olive oil and accompanied by the mint yogurt sauce on the side for dipping.

Cooking and Prep Time

- **Prep Time**: 15 minutes
- **Cook Time**: 15-20 minutes
- **Total Time**: 30-35 minutes

Serving

This recipe serves 4-6 people, with 1-2 chops per serving. The mint yogurt sauce can also be used as a topping or dip for the chops.

Nutrition Information (per serving, based on 6 servings)

- **Calories**: 350
- **Total Fat**: 25g
- **Saturated Fat**: 8g
- **Cholesterol**: 90mg
- **Sodium**: 150mg
- **Total Carbohydrates**: 5g
- **Dietary Fiber**: 1g
- **Protein**: 30g

6.4 Snacks

6.4.1 Hummus with Veggie Sticks

Ingredients

For the Hummus:

- 1 can (400g) chickpeas, drained and rinsed
- 2 tablespoons tahini
- 1-2 garlic cloves, minced (to taste)
- Juice of 1 lemon
- 2 tablespoons olive oil
- Salt to taste
- Water as needed for consistency

For the Veggie Sticks:

- 1 medium carrot, cut into sticks
- 1 cucumber, cut into sticks
- 1 bell pepper (red or yellow), cut into sticks
- 1 celery stalk, cut into sticks

Directions

1. **Prepare the Hummus**: In a food processor, combine the chickpeas, tahini, minced garlic, lemon juice, olive oil, and a pinch of salt. Blend until smooth. If the hummus is too thick, add water, one tablespoon at a time, until you reach your desired consistency.
2. **Taste and Adjust**: Taste the hummus and adjust the seasoning if necessary, adding more salt or lemon juice as desired.
3. **Prepare the Veggies**: While the hummus is blending, wash and cut the vegetables into sticks.

4. **Serve**: Transfer the hummus to a serving bowl and arrange the veggie sticks on a plate around it. Enjoy as a healthy snack or appetizer.

Cooking and Prep Time

- **Prep Time**: 10 minutes
- **Cook Time**: 0 minutes (if using canned chickpeas)
- **Total Time**: 10 minutes

Serving

This recipe serves about 4 people. Each serving can include a generous scoop of hummus along with a variety of vegetable sticks.

Nutritional Information (per serving)

- **Calories**: Approximately 150 kcal
- **Total Fat**: 8g
- **Saturated Fat**: 1g
- **Cholesterol**: 0mg
- **Sodium**: 150mg
- **Total Carbohydrates**: 18g
- **Dietary Fiber**: 5g
- **Sugars**: 2g
- **Protein**: 5g

6.4.2 Apple Slices with Almond Butter

Ingredients

- 1 medium apple (any variety, such as green or red)
- 2 tablespoons almond butter
- Optional toppings:
    - 1 tablespoon sliced almonds
    - 1 tablespoon walnuts
    - 1 tablespoon dark chocolate chips
    - 1 teaspoon cinnamon (for added flavor)

Directions

1. **Prepare the Apple**: Wash the apple thoroughly. Core the apple and slice it into wedges or rounds, depending on your preference.
2. **Spread the Almond Butter**: On a plate, spread almond butter on each apple slice. Use a generous amount to ensure a good balance of flavors.
3. **Add Toppings (Optional)**: If desired, sprinkle sliced almonds, walnuts, or dark chocolate chips on top of the almond butter for added texture and flavor. You can also dust the slices with cinnamon for an extra kick.
4. **Serve**: Arrange the apple slices on a serving plate and enjoy immediately as a healthy snack or dessert.

Cooking and Prep Time

- **Prep Time**: 5 minutes
- **Cook Time**: 0 minutes
- **Total Time**: 5 minutes

Serving

This recipe serves 1 person. You can easily scale it up by multiplying the ingredients for more servings.

Nutritional Information (per serving)

- **Calories**: Approximately 258 kcal (with toppings)
- **Total Fat**: 20g
- **Saturated Fat**: 2g
- **Cholesterol**: 0mg
- **Sodium**: 7mg
- **Total Carbohydrates**: 24g
- **Dietary Fiber**: 4g
- **Sugars**: 10g
- **Protein**: 6g
- **Calcium**: 34% of Daily Value
- **Iron**: 19% of Daily Value

6.4.3 Greek Yogurt with Honey and Nuts

Ingredients

- **For the Greek Yogurt**:
    - 2 cups full-fat Greek yogurt
    - 3/4 teaspoon vanilla extract (optional)

- **For the Toppings**:
    - 1/2 cup toasted walnuts (or a mix of nuts like almonds and hazelnuts)
    - 1/2 cup high-quality honey (adjust to taste)
    - Optional: Cinnamon for sprinkling

Directions

1. **Toast the Nuts**: In a dry skillet over medium heat, add the walnuts (or your choice of nuts). Toast for about 5-6 minutes, stirring frequently, until they are golden brown and fragrant. Remove from heat and let cool.
2. **Prepare the Yogurt**: In a medium bowl, mix the Greek yogurt with vanilla extract (if using) until well combined.
3. **Assemble the Dish**: Spoon the Greek yogurt into serving bowls. Top each bowl with a generous amount of toasted nuts and drizzle honey over the top.
4. **Add Optional Toppings**: For added flavor, sprinkle a pinch of cinnamon over the dish if desired.
5. **Serve Immediately**: Enjoy your Greek yogurt with honey and nuts right away for the best texture and flavor.

Cooking and Prep Time

- **Prep Time**: 5 minutes
- **Cook Time**: 5-6 minutes (for toasting nuts)
- **Total Time**: 10-11 minutes

Serving

This recipe serves 2-4 people, depending on portion sizes. Each serving can be customized with the amount of honey and nuts according to personal preference.

Nutritional Information (per serving, based on 4 servings)

- **Calories**: Approximately 300 kcal
- **Total Fat**: 10g
- **Saturated Fat**: 1.5g
- **Cholesterol**: 10mg
- **Sodium**: 115mg
- **Total Carbohydrates**: 25g
- **Dietary Fiber**: 1g
- **Sugars**: 20g (from honey)
- **Protein**: 29g

6.4.4 Homemade Trail Mix

Ingredients

- **Nuts** (choose any combination):
    - 1 cup almonds
    - 1 cup walnuts
    - 1 cup cashews
    - 1 cup peanuts

- **Seeds**:
    - 1/2 cup sunflower seeds
    - 1/2 cup pumpkin seeds (pepitas)

- **Dried Fruit**:
    - 1 cup raisins or dried cranberries
    - 1/2 cup dried apricots, chopped
    - 1/2 cup dried cherries or banana chips

- **Sweet Treats (optional)**:
    - 1/2 cup dark chocolate chips or M&M's
    - 1/2 cup yogurt-covered raisins

Directions

1. **Prepare Ingredients**: Gather all your nuts, seeds, dried fruits, and any sweet treats you wish to add.
2. **Mix Together**: In a large mixing bowl, combine the nuts, seeds, dried fruit, and sweet treats. Stir well to ensure an even distribution of all ingredients.
3. **Store**: Transfer the trail mix to an airtight container or resealable bag. Store in a cool, dry place.

4. **Serve**: Enjoy your homemade trail mix as a snack on its own or as a topping for yogurt or oatmeal.

Cooking and Prep Time

- **Prep Time**: 5-10 minutes
- **Cook Time**: 0 minutes (no cooking required)
- **Total Time**: 5-10 minutes

Serving

This recipe yields approximately 4-6 servings, depending on portion size. A typical serving size is about 1/4 cup.

Nutritional Information (per serving, based on 6 servings)

- **Calories**: Approximately 200-250 kcal
- **Total Fat**: 15g
- **Saturated Fat**: 2g
- **Cholesterol**: 0mg
- **Sodium**: 5-10mg
- **Total Carbohydrates**: 20-25g
- **Dietary Fiber**: 3-4g
- **Sugars**: 6-10g (from dried fruit and chocolate)
- **Protein**: 6-8g

6.4.5 Rice Cakes with Avocado

Ingredients

- 2 whole grain rice cakes
- 1 ripe avocado, halved and sliced
- 1 tablespoon olive oil (optional)
- Salt and pepper to taste
- Optional toppings:
    - Sliced tomatoes
    - Crumbled feta cheese
    - Chopped fresh herbs (such as cilantro or basil)
    - Red pepper flakes

Directions

1. **Toast the rice cakes**: If desired, lightly toast the rice cakes to add a crispier texture. You can do this in a toaster oven or regular oven preheated to 350°F for 2-3 minutes.
2. **Prepare the avocado**: Slice the avocado in half lengthwise and remove the pit. Scoop out the flesh and slice it into thin strips or chunks.
3. **Assemble the rice cakes**: Place the toasted rice cakes on a plate or cutting board. Drizzle with a small amount of olive oil if desired. Top each rice cake with sliced avocado, spreading it out evenly.
4. **Season and add toppings**: Season the avocado with salt and pepper to taste. Add any desired toppings, such as sliced tomatoes, crumbled feta cheese, chopped fresh herbs, or a sprinkle of red pepper flakes.
5. **Serve immediately**: Enjoy your rice cakes with avocado as a quick and satisfying snack or light meal.

Cooking and Prep Time

- **Prep Time**: 5 minutes

- **Cook Time**: 2-3 minutes (if toasting rice cakes)
- **Total Time**: 7-8 minutes

Serving

This recipe makes 2 servings, with each serving consisting of 1 rice cake topped with half an avocado.

Nutritional Information (per serving)

- **Calories**: Approximately 200 kcal
- **Total Fat**: 13g
- **Saturated Fat**: 2g
- **Cholesterol**: 0mg
- **Sodium**: 5mg
- **Total Carbohydrates**: 19g
- **Dietary Fiber**: 7g
- **Sugars**: 1g
- **Protein**: 3g

6.4.6 Cucumber and Cream Cheese Bites

Ingredients

- **For the Cream Cheese Mixture**:
    - 4 ounces cream cheese, softened
    - 2 tablespoons mayonnaise
    - 1 tablespoon fresh dill, minced (plus extra for garnish)
    - 1 tablespoon chives, chopped (optional)
    - 1 teaspoon lemon juice (optional)
    - Salt and pepper to taste

- **For the Cucumber**:
    - 1-2 cucumbers, sliced into ½ inch rounds

- **Optional Toppings**:
    - Cherry tomatoes, halved
    - Sliced olives
    - Smoked salmon
    - Everything bagel seasoning

Directions

1. **Prepare the Cucumber**: Wash the cucumbers and slice them into ½ inch thick rounds. If desired, you can pat the cucumber slices dry with a paper towel to remove excess moisture.
2. **Make the Cream Cheese Mixture**: In a medium bowl, combine the softened cream cheese, mayonnaise, minced dill, chives (if using), lemon juice (if using), and a pinch of salt and pepper. Mix until smooth and creamy.

3. **Assemble the Bites**: Place the cucumber rounds on a serving platter. Using a spoon or piping bag, dollop or pipe the cream cheese mixture onto each cucumber slice.
4. **Add Toppings**: If desired, top each cream cheese-filled cucumber with additional garnishes such as a cherry tomato half, a slice of olive, or a sprinkle of everything bagel seasoning.
5. **Serve**: Enjoy immediately or refrigerate until ready to serve. These bites are best enjoyed fresh.

Cooking and Prep Time

- **Prep Time**: 10 minutes
- **Cook Time**: 0 minutes (no cooking required)
- **Total Time**: 10 minutes

Serving

This recipe yields approximately 10-12 cucumber bites, depending on the size of the cucumber slices. It can easily be doubled or tripled for larger gatherings.

Nutritional Information (per bite, based on 12 servings)

- **Calories**: Approximately 30 kcal
- **Total Fat**: 2g
- **Saturated Fat**: 1g
- **Cholesterol**: 5mg
- **Sodium**: 50mg
- **Total Carbohydrates**: 2g
- **Dietary Fiber**: 0g
- **Sugars**: 1g
- **Protein**: 1g

6.4.7 Baked Sweet Potato Chips

Ingredients

- **For the Cream Cheese Mixture**:
    - 4 ounces cream cheese, softened
    - 2 tablespoons mayonnaise
    - 1 tablespoon fresh dill, minced (plus extra for garnish)
    - 1 tablespoon chives, chopped (optional)
    - 1 teaspoon lemon juice (optional)
    - Salt and pepper to taste

- **For the Cucumber**:
    - 1-2 cucumbers, sliced into ½ inch rounds

- **Optional Toppings**:
    - Cherry tomatoes, halved
    - Sliced olives
    - Smoked salmon
    - Everything bagel seasoning

Directions

1. **Prepare the Cucumber**: Wash the cucumbers and slice them into ½ inch thick rounds. If desired, you can pat the cucumber slices dry with a paper towel to remove excess moisture.
2. **Make the Cream Cheese Mixture**: In a medium bowl, combine the softened cream cheese, mayonnaise, minced dill, chives (if using), lemon juice (if using), and a pinch of salt and pepper. Mix until smooth and creamy.

3. **Assemble the Bites**: Place the cucumber rounds on a serving platter. Using a spoon or piping bag, dollop or pipe the cream cheese mixture onto each cucumber slice.
4. **Add Toppings**: If desired, top each cream cheese-filled cucumber with additional garnishes such as a cherry tomato half, a slice of olive, or a sprinkle of everything bagel seasoning.
5. **Serve**: Enjoy immediately or refrigerate until ready to serve. These bites are best enjoyed fresh.

Cooking and Prep Time

- **Prep Time**: 10 minutes
- **Cook Time**: 0 minutes (no cooking required)
- **Total Time**: 10 minutes

Serving

This recipe yields approximately 10-12 cucumber bites, depending on the size of the cucumber slices. It can easily be doubled or tripled for larger gatherings.

Nutritional Information (per bite, based on 12 servings)

- **Calories**: Approximately 30 kcal
- **Total Fat**: 2g
- **Saturated Fat**: 1g
- **Cholesterol**: 5mg
- **Sodium**: 50mg
- **Total Carbohydrates**: 2g
- **Dietary Fiber**: 0g
- **Sugars**: 1g
- **Protein**: 1g

6.4.8 Protein Balls

Ingredients

- **Base Ingredients**:
    - 1 cup rolled oats
    - 1/2 cup nut butter (e.g., peanut butter, almond butter, or sunflower seed butter)
    - 1/4 cup honey or maple syrup
    - 1/2 cup protein powder (your choice of flavor)

- **Optional Mix-ins**:
    - 1/4 cup chocolate chips or mini chocolate chips
    - 1/4 cup chopped nuts (e.g., almonds, walnuts)
    - 1/4 cup dried fruit (e.g., raisins, cranberries)
    - 1 tablespoon chia seeds or flaxseeds
    - 1 teaspoon vanilla extract (for added flavor)

Directions

1. **Mix the Base Ingredients**: In a large mixing bowl, combine the rolled oats, nut butter, honey (or maple syrup), and protein powder. Stir until well combined. The mixture will be thick and sticky.
2. **Add Optional Mix-ins**: If desired, fold in chocolate chips, nuts, dried fruit, chia seeds, or any other mix-ins you prefer.
3. **Form the Balls**: Using your hands or a cookie scoop, form the mixture into small balls (about 1 inch in diameter).
4. **Chill**: Place the protein balls on a lined baking sheet or plate and refrigerate for at least 30 minutes to firm up.
5. **Store**: Once firm, transfer the protein balls to an airtight container. They can be stored in the refrigerator for up to 2 weeks or frozen for up to 3 months.

Cooking and Prep Time

- **Prep Time**: 10 minutes
- **Chill Time**: 30 minutes
- **Total Time**: 40 minutes

Serving

This recipe yields approximately 12-15 protein balls, depending on the size. Each serving can be 1-2 balls, making it a great snack option for sharing.

Nutritional Information (per protein ball, based on 15 servings)

- **Calories**: Approximately 100 kcal
- **Total Fat**: 5g
- **Saturated Fat**: 1g
- **Cholesterol**: 0mg
- **Sodium**: 50mg
- **Total Carbohydrates**: 10g
- **Dietary Fiber**: 2g
- **Sugars**: 3g
- **Protein**: 5g

6.4.9 Edamame with Sea Salt

Ingredients

- **Edamame**: 2 cups frozen edamame in pods (or fresh if available)
- **Water**: 6 cups
- **Sea Salt**: 1 tablespoon (adjust to taste)

Directions

1. **Boil Water**: In a large pot, bring 6 cups of water to a boil. Add 1 tablespoon of sea salt to the water.
2. **Cook Edamame**: Once the water is boiling, add the frozen (or fresh) edamame pods. Cook for about 5 minutes, or until the pods are tender and easily release from their shells.
3. **Drain**: After cooking, drain the edamame in a colander and let them cool for a minute.
4. **Season**: While the edamame is still warm, sprinkle additional sea salt over the pods to taste. Toss gently to ensure the salt is evenly distributed.
5. **Serve**: Place the edamame in a serving bowl. Serve warm or at room temperature as a snack or appetizer. To eat, simply pop the beans out of the pods with your mouth and discard the shells.

Cooking and Prep Time

- **Prep Time**: 5 minutes
- **Cook Time**: 5 minutes
- **Total Time**: 10 minutes

Serving

This recipe serves approximately 2-4 people, depending on portion sizes. Each serving can include about 1 cup of cooked edamame pods.

Nutritional Information (per serving, based on 4 servings)

- **Calories**: Approximately 120 kcal

- **Total Fat**: 4g
- **Saturated Fat**: 0.5g
- **Cholesterol**: 0mg
- **Sodium**: 300mg (with added salt)
- **Total Carbohydrates**: 14g
- **Dietary Fiber**: 5g
- **Sugars**: 2g
- **Protein**: 11g

6.4.10 Stuffed Dates

Ingredients

- **For the Stuffed Dates**:
    - 12 ounces pitted Medjool dates
    - 4 ounces goat cheese, softened
    - 1/3 cup finely chopped walnuts
    - 2 teaspoons minced fresh rosemary
    - 1 teaspoon orange zest
    - 2 teaspoons fresh orange juice
    - 1/4 teaspoon ground cinnamon
    - 1/4 teaspoon sea salt
    - 3 tablespoons extra-virgin olive oil

- **For Drizzling** (optional):
    - Hot honey or regular honey

Directions

1. **Preheat Oven**: Preheat your oven to 375°F (190°C).
2. **Prepare Dates**: Use a small sharp knife to slice each date lengthwise without cutting all the way through. Gently open the date and fill it with 1 to 2 teaspoons of goat cheese.
3. **Mix Topping**: In a small bowl, combine the chopped walnuts, minced rosemary, orange zest, orange juice, ground cinnamon, sea salt, and olive oil. Mix well to combine.
4. **Stuff and Arrange**: Spoon the walnut mixture over the stuffed dates and arrange them in a baking dish.
5. **Roast**: Bake the dates in the preheated oven for about 15 minutes, or until they are heated through and slightly golden.

6. **Serve**: Remove from the oven and let cool for a few minutes. Drizzle with hot honey if desired, then transfer to a serving platter. Serve warm.

Cooking and Prep Time

- **Prep Time**: 15 minutes
- **Cook Time**: 15 minutes
- **Total Time**: 30 minutes

Serving

This recipe yields approximately 8 servings, with each serving consisting of 2-3 stuffed dates.

Nutritional Information (per serving, based on 8 servings)

- **Calories**: Approximately 150 kcal
- **Total Fat**: 10g
- **Saturated Fat**: 3g
- **Cholesterol**: 10mg
- **Sodium**: 100mg
- **Total Carbohydrates**: 15g
- **Dietary Fiber**: 2g
- **Sugars**: 10g
- **Protein**: 3g

6.4.11 Chia Seed Pudding

Ingredients

- **Base Ingredients**:
    - 4 tablespoons chia seeds
    - 1 cup milk (any type: almond, coconut, oat, or dairy)
    - 1/2 tablespoon maple syrup or honey (optional, adjust to taste)
    - 1/4 teaspoon vanilla extract (optional)

- **Optional Toppings**:
    - Fresh fruits (berries, bananas, mango)
    - Granola or nuts
    - Coconut flakes
    - Nut butter
    - Cinnamon or cocoa powder

Directions

1. **Combine Ingredients**: In a bowl or a mason jar, mix together the chia seeds, milk, maple syrup (or honey), and vanilla extract (if using). Stir well to ensure the chia seeds are evenly distributed.
2. **Let it Sit**: Allow the mixture to sit for about 5 minutes. Stir again to break up any clumps of chia seeds that may have formed.
3. **Refrigerate**: Cover the bowl or jar and place it in the refrigerator. Let the pudding set for at least 1-2 hours, or preferably overnight. The chia seeds will absorb the liquid and create a thick, pudding-like consistency.
4. **Serve**: Once the pudding has thickened, give it a good stir. Serve it in bowls or jars, and add your favorite toppings such as fresh fruits, granola, or nuts.

Cooking and Prep Time

- **Prep Time**: 10 minutes

- **Chill Time**: 1-2 hours (or overnight)
- **Total Time**: 1 hour 10 minutes to overnight

Serving

This recipe yields about 2 servings, with each serving being approximately 1/2 cup of chia seed pudding.

Nutritional Information (per serving, based on 2 servings)

- **Calories**: Approximately 170 kcal
- **Total Fat**: 9g
- **Saturated Fat**: 1g
- **Cholesterol**: 0mg
- **Sodium**: 91mg
- **Total Carbohydrates**: 16g
- **Dietary Fiber**: 13g
- **Sugars**: 3g (with maple syrup)
- **Protein**: 7g

6.4.12 Celery Sticks with Peanut Butter

Ingredients

- 4-6 celery stalks, washed and cut into 4-inch pieces (about 3 pieces per stalk)
- 1/2 cup creamy or crunchy peanut butter
- Optional toppings:
  - Raisins or dried cranberries
  - Chopped nuts
  - Chocolate chips

Directions

1. Wash the celery stalks and cut them into 4-inch pieces, creating about 3 pieces per stalk.
2. Spread about 1-2 teaspoons of peanut butter into the "furrow" of each celery stick, filling it generously.
3. If desired, top the peanut butter-filled celery sticks with raisins, dried cranberries, chopped nuts, or chocolate chips for added flavor and texture.
4. Arrange the prepared celery sticks on a plate or in a container and serve immediately or refrigerate until ready to enjoy.

Cooking and Prep Time

- **Prep Time**: 10 minutes
- **Cook Time**: 0 minutes (no cooking required)
- **Total Time**: 10 minutes

Serving

This recipe yields approximately 12 celery sticks, with each serving consisting of 1-2 sticks, depending on appetite and portion size preferences.

Nutritional Information (per serving, based on 12 servings)

- **Calories**: Approximately 100 kcal

- **Total Fat**: 8g
- **Saturated Fat**: 1g
- **Cholesterol**: 0mg
- **Sodium**: 100mg
- **Total Carbohydrates**: 5g
- **Dietary Fiber**: 2g
- **Sugars**: 2g
- **Protein**: 4g

6.4.13 Homemade Popcorn

Ingredients

- **3 tablespoons** coconut oil or olive oil
- **1/2 cup** popcorn kernels
- **1/4 teaspoon** salt (or to taste)
- **Optional Toppings**:
    - Melted butter or coconut oil
    - Grated parmesan cheese
    - Chili powder or paprika
    - Garlic powder
    - Dried herbs (such as rosemary or thyme)

Directions

1. **In a large pot with a tight-fitting lid**, heat the coconut oil or olive oil over medium heat.
2. **Add 3 popcorn kernels to the pot** and cover. Wait for the kernels to pop, which will indicate that the oil is hot enough.
3. **Once the 3 kernels have popped**, add the remaining 1/2 cup of popcorn kernels in an even layer. Cover the pot and keep it on the heat.
4. **Once the popping starts**, gently shake the pot back and forth to prevent burning. Continue shaking until the popping slows to about 2-3 seconds between pops.
5. **Remove the pot from heat** and transfer the popped popcorn to a large bowl.
6. **Season with salt** and any desired toppings. Toss to evenly distribute the seasonings.
7. **Serve the popcorn warm** and enjoy!

Cooking and Prep Time

- **Prep Time**: 5 minutes

- **Cook Time**: 5-7 minutes
- **Total Time**: 10-12 minutes

Serving

This recipe yields approximately 4 cups of popped popcorn, which can serve 2-4 people, depending on portion size preferences.

Nutritional Information (per serving, based on 4 servings)

- **Calories**: Approximately 150 kcal
- **Total Fat**: 10g
- **Saturated Fat**: 8g
- **Cholesterol**: 0mg
- **Sodium**: 200mg
- **Total Carbohydrates**: 15g
- **Dietary Fiber**: 3g
- **Sugars**: 0g
- **Protein**: 2g

6.4.14 Fruit Smoothie

Ingredients

- **Base Ingredients**:
    - 1 cup fresh or frozen fruit (such as bananas, berries, mangoes, or peaches)
    - 1 cup milk (dairy or plant-based, such as almond, coconut, or oat milk)
    - 1/2 cup Greek yogurt (optional, for added creaminess and protein)
    - 1 tablespoon honey or maple syrup (optional, for sweetness)
    - 1/2 teaspoon vanilla extract (optional)

- **Optional Add-ins**:
    - 1 tablespoon chia seeds or flaxseeds (for added fiber and omega-3s)
    - 1 scoop protein powder (for extra protein)
    - A handful of spinach or kale (for added nutrients without altering the flavor)

Directions

1. **Prepare the Ingredients**: If using fresh fruit, wash and chop it into smaller pieces. If using frozen fruit, there's no need to thaw it.
2. **Blend**: In a blender, combine the fruit, milk, Greek yogurt (if using), honey or maple syrup (if desired), and vanilla extract. If adding any optional ingredients, include them as well.
3. **Blend Until Smooth**: Blend on high speed until the mixture is smooth and creamy. If the smoothie is too thick, add a little more milk until you reach your desired consistency.
4. **Taste and Adjust**: Taste the smoothie and adjust sweetness if needed by adding more honey or syrup.
5. **Serve**: Pour the smoothie into a glass and enjoy immediately. You can also garnish with additional fruit or seeds on top if desired.

Cooking and Prep Time

- **Prep Time**: 5 minutes
- **Cook Time**: 0 minutes (no cooking required)
- **Total Time**: 5 minutes

Serving

This recipe yields approximately 2 servings, with each serving being about 1 cup of smoothie.

Nutritional Information (per serving, based on 2 servings)

- **Calories**: Approximately 180-250 kcal (depending on ingredients used)
- **Total Fat**: 3-8g (depending on milk and yogurt used)
- **Saturated Fat**: 1-3g
- **Cholesterol**: 5-15mg (if using dairy yogurt)
- **Sodium**: 50-100mg
- **Total Carbohydrates**: 30-40g
- **Dietary Fiber**: 3-5g
- **Sugars**: 15-25g (natural sugars from fruit and added sweeteners)
- **Protein**: 5-10g (depending on yogurt and protein powder)

6.4.15 Spiced Nuts

Ingredients

- **Nuts**:
  - 2 cups mixed nuts (such as almonds, walnuts, pecans, and cashews)

- **Spice Mixture**:
  - 1 tablespoon olive oil
  - 1 teaspoon sea salt
  - 1 teaspoon smoked paprika
  - 1/2 teaspoon garlic powder
  - 1/2 teaspoon onion powder
  - 1/2 teaspoon cayenne pepper (adjust to taste)
  - 1/2 teaspoon ground cumin
  - 1/2 teaspoon dried thyme or rosemary (optional)

- **Sweetener (optional)**:
  - 1 tablespoon maple syrup or honey (for a sweet-spicy version)

Directions

1. **Preheat Oven**: Preheat your oven to 350°F (175°C).
2. **Prepare the Nuts**: In a large mixing bowl, combine the mixed nuts.
3. **Make the Spice Mixture**: In a small bowl, whisk together the olive oil, sea salt, smoked paprika, garlic powder, onion powder, cayenne pepper, ground cumin, and thyme or rosemary (if using). If you prefer a sweet version, add the maple syrup or honey to the mixture.
4. **Coat the Nuts**: Pour the spice mixture over the nuts and stir until all the nuts are evenly coated.

5. **Spread on Baking Sheet**: Spread the coated nuts in a single layer on a baking sheet lined with parchment paper.

6. **Bake**: Bake in the preheated oven for about 15-20 minutes, stirring halfway through, until the nuts are golden brown and fragrant. Keep an eye on them to prevent burning.

7. **Cool and Serve**: Remove from the oven and let the spiced nuts cool completely. Once cooled, transfer them to an airtight container for storage or serve immediately.

Cooking and Prep Time

- **Prep Time**: 10 minutes
- **Cook Time**: 15-20 minutes
- **Total Time**: 25-30 minutes

Serving

This recipe yields approximately 4 servings, with each serving being about 1/2 cup of spiced nuts.

Nutritional Information (per serving, based on 4 servings)

- **Calories**: Approximately 200 kcal
- **Total Fat**: 18g
- **Saturated Fat**: 2g
- **Cholesterol**: 0mg
- **Sodium**: 200mg
- **Total Carbohydrates**: 8g
- **Dietary Fiber**: 3g
- **Sugars**: 1g (without sweetener)
- **Protein**: 5g

6.5 Desserts

6.5.1 Berry Coconut Crumble

Ingredients

- 300-350g mixed berries (raspberries, blueberries, blackberries, etc.), fresh or frozen
- 2-3 tbsp sugar or honey, to taste
- 1 cup rolled oats
- 1/2 cup shredded coconut
- 3-4 tbsp butter or coconut oil, melted
- 1/4 tsp cinnamon (optional)

Instructions

1. Preheat oven to 350°F (180°C).
2. In a bowl, gently mix the berries with 1-2 tbsp of the sugar or honey. Transfer to a greased baking dish or 4-6 ramekins.
3. In another bowl, combine the oats, coconut, remaining sugar, cinnamon (if using), and melted butter/coconut oil. Mix until well combined.
4. Sprinkle the oat-coconut mixture evenly over the berries.
5. Bake for 20-25 minutes, until the topping is golden brown and the berries are bubbling.
6. Let cool for 10 minutes before serving warm, with a scoop of vanilla ice cream, yogurt, or whipped cream if desired.

Prep Time: 10 minutes

Cook Time: 20-25 minutes

Servings: 4-6

Nutrition (per serving, approximate):

- Calories: 250-300
- Carbohydrates: 30-35g

- Fiber: 5-7g
- Protein: 3-5g
- Fat: 12-15g

6.5.2 Almond Flour Brownies

Ingredients

- 1 ½ cups blanched almond flour
- ¾ cup unsweetened cocoa powder
- 1 ¾ cups granulated sugar (or sweetener of choice)
- 1 teaspoon baking powder
- ½ teaspoon salt
- 5 tablespoons unsalted butter, melted (or coconut oil for dairy-free)
- 3 large eggs, room temperature
- 1 teaspoon vanilla extract
- ½ cup chocolate chips (optional)

Directions

1. **Preheat the Oven**: Preheat your oven to 350°F (180°C). Line an 8x8-inch baking pan with parchment paper.
2. **Mix Dry Ingredients**: In a medium bowl, whisk together the almond flour, cocoa powder, baking powder, and salt until well combined.
3. **Combine Wet Ingredients**: In a separate large bowl, whisk together the melted butter, sugar, eggs, and vanilla extract until smooth.
4. **Combine Mixtures**: Gradually add the dry ingredients to the wet ingredients, mixing until fully incorporated. If using, fold in the chocolate chips.
5. **Bake**: Pour the batter into the prepared pan, spreading it evenly. Bake for 33 to 38 minutes, or until a toothpick inserted into the center comes out clean or with a few moist crumbs.
6. **Cool and Serve**: Allow the brownies to cool in the pan for about 15-20 minutes before lifting them out and slicing into squares.

Cooking and Prep Time

- **Prep Time**: 10 minutes
- **Cook Time**: 35-38 minutes

- **Total Time**: Approximately 50-55 minutes

Servings

- Makes about 12 brownies.

Nutrition (per brownie, approximate)

- Calories: 200-220
- Carbohydrates: 25g
- Fiber: 3g
- Protein: 4g
- Fat: 10g
- Sugar: 15g

6.5.3 Chocolate Chia Pudding

Ingredients

- 1/2 cup chia seeds
- 1 ½ cups unsweetened almond milk (or any milk of choice)
- 1/4 cup unsweetened cocoa powder
- 3-5 tablespoons maple syrup (to taste)
- 1/2 teaspoon vanilla extract
- A pinch of sea salt

Directions

1. **Combine Ingredients**: In a medium mixing bowl, whisk together the almond milk, cocoa powder, maple syrup, vanilla extract, and salt until smooth.
2. **Add Chia Seeds**: Stir in the chia seeds, ensuring they are evenly distributed throughout the mixture.
3. **Rest and Thicken**: Let the mixture sit for about 10 minutes, then whisk again to break up any clumps of chia seeds. This helps ensure even thickening.
4. **Chill**: Cover the bowl or transfer the mixture to individual jars. Refrigerate for at least 4 hours, or overnight for the best results. The pudding will thicken as it chills.
5. **Serve**: Once thickened, stir the pudding again before serving. Top with your favorite fruits, nuts, or granola if desired.

Cooking and Prep Time

- **Prep Time**: 10 minutes
- **Chill Time**: 4 hours (or overnight)
- **Total Time**: Approximately 4 hours 10 minutes

Servings

- Makes about 4 servings.

Nutrition (per serving, approximate)

- Calories: 186
- Carbohydrates: 26g
- Protein: 5g
- Fat: 9g
- Saturated Fat: 1g
- Fiber: 10g
- Sugar: 12g

6.5.4 Baked Apples with Cinnamon

Ingredients

- 5-6 large apples (Granny Smith, Honeycrisp, or Fuji recommended)
- 1 tablespoon lemon juice
- ¼ cup light brown sugar
- 1 tablespoon granulated sugar
- 2 teaspoons ground cinnamon
- 2 teaspoons cornstarch
- 2 tablespoons unsalted butter, cut into small pieces

Directions

1. **Preheat the Oven**: Preheat your oven to 375°F (190°C).
2. **Prepare the Apples**: Peel, core, and slice the apples. Place them in a 9x13-inch baking dish.
3. **Mix Ingredients**: In a large bowl, combine the lemon juice, brown sugar, granulated sugar, cinnamon, and cornstarch. Mix well, then pour this mixture over the sliced apples. Toss to coat the apples evenly.
4. **Arrange in Dish**: Spread the apple mixture evenly in the baking dish and dot with pieces of butter on top.
5. **Bake**: Cover the dish with foil and bake for 30-40 minutes. Stir the apples every 10-15 minutes to ensure even cooking. The apples should be tender when done.
6. **Cool and Serve**: Once baked, let the apples cool for about 10 minutes before serving. They can be enjoyed warm, plain, or with a scoop of vanilla ice cream.

Cooking and Prep Time

- **Prep Time**: 15 minutes
- **Cook Time**: 30-40 minutes
- **Total Time**: Approximately 55 minutes

Servings

- Serves about 6 people.

Nutrition (per serving, approximate)

- Calories: 160
- Carbohydrates: 36g
- Fiber: 5g
- Protein: 1g
- Fat: 4g
- Sugar: 20g

6.5.5 Avocado Chocolate Mousse

Ingredients

- 2 ripe avocados
- 1/2 cup unsweetened cocoa powder
- 1/4 cup maple syrup (or honey)
- 1/4 cup unsweetened almond milk (or coconut milk)
- 1 teaspoon vanilla extract
- 1/4 teaspoon sea salt

Instructions

1. **Scoop the flesh** of the avocados into a food processor or high-powered blender.
2. **Add the cocoa powder, maple syrup, almond milk, vanilla extract, and salt**. Blend until completely smooth and creamy, scraping down the sides as needed.
3. **Transfer the mousse** to individual serving dishes or one larger serving bowl.
4. **Refrigerate for at least 30 minutes** before serving to allow the flavors to meld and the texture to thicken.
5. **Serve chilled**, garnished with fresh berries, toasted coconut, or a dusting of cocoa powder if desired.

Prep Time: 10 minutes

Cook Time: 0 minutes

Total Time: 10 minutes + 30 minutes chilling

Servings: 4

Nutrition (per serving):

- Calories: 220
- Fat: 13g
- Carbohydrates: 26g
- Fiber: 9g
- Protein: 4g

6.5.6 Frozen Banana Bites

Ingredients

- 3-4 medium-sized ripe bananas
- 1 cup chocolate chips (semi-sweet or dark)
- 1 tablespoon coconut oil (optional, for smoother chocolate)
- Sea salt (optional, for topping)

Directions

1. **Prepare the Bananas**: Peel the bananas and slice them into 1/2-inch thick rounds. Arrange the slices in a single layer on a baking sheet lined with parchment paper.
2. **Freeze the Banana Slices**: Place the baking sheet in the freezer and freeze the banana slices for about 30 minutes, or until firm.
3. **Melt the Chocolate**: In a microwave-safe bowl, combine the chocolate chips and coconut oil. Microwave in 30-second intervals, stirring in between, until the chocolate is completely melted and smooth.
4. **Dip the Bananas**: Remove the frozen banana slices from the freezer. Using a fork, dip each slice into the melted chocolate, ensuring it is fully coated. Allow any excess chocolate to drip off.
5. **Return to the Baking Sheet**: Place the chocolate-covered banana slices back on the parchment-lined baking sheet. If desired, sprinkle a pinch of sea salt on top of each piece before the chocolate sets.
6. **Freeze Again**: Return the baking sheet to the freezer for an additional 30 minutes to allow the chocolate to harden.
7. **Serve**: Once the chocolate is set, transfer the banana bites to an airtight container and store in the freezer until ready to serve.

Cooking and Prep Time

- **Prep Time**: 15 minutes
- **Freezing Time**: 1 hour (30 minutes for bananas + 30 minutes for chocolate)

- **Total Time**: Approximately 1 hour 15 minutes

Servings

- Makes about 20-30 bites, depending on the size of the banana slices.

Nutrition (per bite, approximate)

- Calories: 50
- Fat: 3g
- Carbohydrates: 6g
- Fiber: 1g
- Protein: 1g
- Sugar: 3g

6.5.7 Coconut Macaroons

Ingredients

- 14 oz. sweetened flaked coconut (about 396g)
- 1 cup sweetened condensed milk (about 380g)
- 1 teaspoon vanilla extract
- 2 large egg whites
- A pinch of salt
- 1/2 cup chocolate chips (optional, for dipping)

Directions

1. **Preheat the Oven**: Preheat your oven to 325°F (162°C). Line two baking sheets with parchment paper.
2. **Mix Coconut Ingredients**: In a large bowl, combine the sweetened coconut, sweetened condensed milk, and vanilla extract. Mix until well combined.
3. **Beat Egg Whites**: In a separate bowl, beat the egg whites and a pinch of salt using a hand mixer or stand mixer until stiff peaks form. This means that when you lift the beaters out, the egg whites will hold their shape.
4. **Fold Mixtures Together**: Gently fold the beaten egg whites into the coconut mixture. Be careful not to deflate the egg whites; use a spatula to incorporate them until just combined.
5. **Scoop and Bake**: Using a mini ice cream scoop or two spoons, drop heaping tablespoons of the mixture onto the prepared baking sheets, spacing them about 1 inch apart. Bake for 23-26 minutes, or until the tops are lightly golden.
6. **Cool**: Once baked, let the macaroons cool on the baking sheets for about 5 minutes before transferring them to a wire rack to cool completely.
7. **Optional Chocolate Dip**: If desired, melt the chocolate chips in a microwave-safe bowl in 30-second intervals, stirring until smooth. Dip the bottoms of the cooled macaroons into the melted chocolate and return them to

the parchment-lined baking sheets. Refrigerate for about 10 minutes to allow the chocolate to set.

Cooking and Prep Time

- **Prep Time**: 15 minutes
- **Cook Time**: 25-30 minutes
- **Total Time**: Approximately 45-60 minutes

Servings

- Makes about 20-24 macaroons.

Nutrition (per macaroon, approximate)

- Calories: 120
- Fat: 6g
- Carbohydrates: 15g
- Fiber: 1g
- Protein: 2g
- Sugar: 10g

6.5.8 Pumpkin Spice Muffins

Ingredients

- 1 cup all-purpose flour
- 1/2 teaspoon baking powder
- 1/2 teaspoon baking soda
- 1/2 teaspoon ground cinnamon
- 1/2 teaspoon pumpkin pie spice
- 1/4 teaspoon salt
- 1/4 cup unsalted butter, melted (or a neutral oil)
- 1/2 cup pumpkin puree (canned or homemade)
- 1/3 cup brown sugar, packed
- 1 large egg
- 1/2 teaspoon vanilla extract
- 1 tablespoon turbinado or granulated sugar (for sprinkling on top)

Directions

1. **Preheat the Oven**: Preheat your oven to 425°F (220°C). Line a muffin tin with paper liners or grease it lightly.
2. **Mix Dry Ingredients**: In a medium bowl, whisk together the flour, baking powder, baking soda, cinnamon, pumpkin pie spice, and salt until well combined.
3. **Combine Wet Ingredients**: In a large bowl, whisk together the melted butter, pumpkin puree, brown sugar, egg, and vanilla extract until smooth.
4. **Combine Mixtures**: Add the dry ingredients to the wet ingredients and stir until just combined. Be careful not to overmix; a few lumps are okay.
5. **Scoop Batter**: Using a scoop or spoon, fill each muffin cup about 3/4 full with the batter. Sprinkle a little turbinado or granulated sugar on top of each muffin for a crunchy finish.

6. **Bake**: Bake in the preheated oven for 5 minutes at 425°F, then reduce the temperature to 350°F (175°C) and continue baking for an additional 12-14 minutes, or until a toothpick inserted into the center comes out clean.
7. **Cool**: Allow the muffins to cool in the pan for about 5 minutes, then transfer them to a wire rack to cool completely.

Cooking and Prep Time

- **Prep Time**: 10 minutes
- **Cook Time**: 17-19 minutes
- **Total Time**: Approximately 30 minutes

Servings

- Makes about 6 muffins.

Nutrition (per muffin, approximate)

- Calories: 150
- Fat: 6g
- Carbohydrates: 22g
- Fiber: 1g
- Protein: 2g
- Sugar: 8g

6.5.9 Fruit Sorbet

Ingredients

- **Option 1 (1-Ingredient Sorbet)**:
    - 2 cups frozen fruit of choice (e.g., mixed berries, mango, or banana)

- **Option 2 (2-Ingredient Sorbet)**:
    - 3 cups frozen fruit of choice (e.g., strawberries, pineapple, or peaches)
    - 4 tablespoons coconut milk (or milk of choice)

Directions

1. **Prepare the Fruit**: If using fresh fruit, slice and freeze it for at least 4 hours or until solid. For frozen fruit, ensure it's ready to use.
2. **Blend Ingredients**:
    - **For Option 1**: Place the frozen fruit in a high-speed blender or food processor. Blend until smooth and creamy, stopping to scrape down the sides as needed.
    - **For Option 2**: Add the frozen fruit and coconut milk to the blender or food processor. Blend until smooth, scraping down the sides as necessary.

3. **Taste and Adjust**: If desired, you can add a sweetener like maple syrup or honey to taste, especially if the fruit isn't sweet enough.
4. **Serve or Store**:
    - Serve immediately for a soft-serve texture.
    - For a firmer texture, transfer the sorbet to an airtight container and freeze for at least 1-2 hours before serving.

5. **Optional**: Garnish with fresh fruit, mint leaves, or a sprinkle of coconut flakes before serving.

Cooking and Prep Time

- **Prep Time**: 5 minutes
- **Freezing Time**: 4 hours (if using fresh fruit)
- **Total Time**: Approximately 5 minutes + freezing time

Servings

- Makes about 4-6 servings, depending on portion size.

Nutrition (per serving, approximate for 1-Ingredient Sorbet)

- Calories: 80
- Fat: 1g
- Carbohydrates: 20g
- Fiber: 2g
- Protein: 1g
- Sugar: 15g

6.5.10 Date and Nut Energy Balls

Ingredients

- 1 cup Medjool dates, pitted
- 1 cup mixed nuts (such as almonds, walnuts, pecans)
- 1/2 cup rolled oats
- 2 tablespoons unsweetened shredded coconut
- 1 tablespoon almond butter
- 1 teaspoon vanilla extract
- 1/4 teaspoon sea salt

Instructions

1. **Soak the dates**: If the dates are firm, place them in a bowl and cover with hot water. Let soak for 10-15 minutes to soften. Drain and pat dry.
2. **Process the ingredients**: In a food processor, combine the soaked dates, nuts, oats, coconut, almond butter, vanilla and salt. Process until the mixture starts to stick together, about 1-2 minutes, scraping down the sides as needed.
3. **Form the balls**: Scoop out tablespoon-sized portions of the mixture and roll into balls with your hands. Place on a parchment-lined baking sheet.
4. **Chill**: Refrigerate the energy balls for at least 30 minutes to help them firm up.
5. **Serve**: Enjoy the chilled energy balls as a healthy snack. Store leftovers in an airtight container in the fridge for up to 1 week or in the freezer for up to 3 months.

Prep Time: 15 minutes

Chill Time: 30 minutes

Total Time: 45 minutes

Servings: 12-15 balls

Nutrition (per ball):

- Calories: 120

- Fat: 6g
- Carbohydrates: 16g
- Fiber: 3g
- Protein: 2g

6.5.11 Greek Yogurt Parfait

Ingredients

- 2 cups plain Greek yogurt
- 2 tablespoons honey or maple syrup (optional)
- 2 cups mixed berries (such as strawberries, blueberries, raspberries)
- 1 cup granola

Instructions

1. **If sweetening the yogurt**, stir in the honey or maple syrup until fully incorporated.
2. **In a parfait glass or mason jar**, layer half of the yogurt on the bottom.
3. **Top the yogurt with a layer of berries**, followed by a layer of granola.
4. **Repeat the layers**, ending with a final layer of yogurt.
5. **Refrigerate until ready to serve.**

Prep Time: 10 minutes

Cook Time: 0 minutes

Total Time: 10 minutes

Servings: 4

Nutrition (per serving):

- Calories: 300
- Fat: 8g
- Carbohydrates: 40g
- Fiber: 5g
- Protein: 20g

6.5.12 Apple Cinnamon Oat Bars

Ingredients

- 4 medium apples, peeled and chopped
- 1 cup all-purpose flour
- 1/4 teaspoon salt
- 1/2 teaspoon baking soda
- 1/2 teaspoon ground cinnamon
- 1/2 cup brown sugar, packed
- 1 cup rolled oats
- 1/2 cup unsalted butter, melted
- 2 large eggs
- 1 teaspoon vanilla extract

Directions

1. **Preheat the Oven**: Preheat your oven to 350°F (175°C). Grease a 9x9-inch baking dish.
2. **Prepare the Apples**: Peel and chop the apples into small pieces. Set aside.
3. **Mix Dry Ingredients**: In a medium bowl, combine the flour, salt, baking soda, cinnamon, brown sugar, and oats. Mix well.
4. **Combine Wet Ingredients**: In a separate large bowl, whisk together the melted butter, eggs, and vanilla extract until smooth.
5. **Combine Mixtures**: Gradually add the dry ingredients to the wet ingredients, stirring until just combined. Gently fold in the chopped apples.
6. **Spread in Baking Dish**: Pour the batter into the prepared baking dish and spread it evenly.
7. **Bake**: Bake for 25-30 minutes, or until the edges are golden brown and a toothpick inserted into the center comes out clean.
8. **Cool and Serve**: Allow the bars to cool in the pan for about 10 minutes before cutting into squares. Serve warm or at room temperature.

Cooking and Prep Time

- **Prep Time**: 15 minutes
- **Cook Time**: 25-30 minutes
- **Total Time**: Approximately 45-55 minutes

Servings

- Makes about 12 bars.

Nutrition (per bar, approximate)

- Calories: 180
- Fat: 7g
- Carbohydrates: 27g
- Fiber: 2g
- Protein: 3g
- Sugar: 10g

6.5.13 Raspberry Lemon Bars

Ingredients

For the crust:

- 2 cups all-purpose flour
- 3/4 cup unsalted butter, cubed
- 2/3 cup powdered sugar
- 1/4 teaspoon salt

For the raspberry layer:

- 2 pints fresh raspberries
- 1/4 cup sugar
- 2 tablespoons water
- 4 tablespoons cornstarch

For the lemon filling:

- 4 large eggs
- 1 1/2 cups granulated sugar
- 6 tablespoons all-purpose flour
- 1/2 cup fresh lemon juice (from 2-3 lemons)
- 2 teaspoons lemon zest
- Powdered sugar for dusting (optional)

Directions

1. **Preheat the Oven**: Preheat your oven to 350°F (175°C). Line a 13x9-inch baking pan with foil, allowing some overhang for easy removal, and lightly grease the foil.
2. **Prepare the Raspberry Sauce**: In a small saucepan, combine the raspberries, sugar, and water. Cook over medium heat, stirring frequently, until the mixture is thick and bubbly. Mash any whole berries with the back of a spoon. Once thickened, remove from heat and keep warm.

3. **Make the Crust**: In a food processor, combine the flour, powdered sugar, and salt. Add the cubed butter and pulse until the mixture resembles coarse sand. Press the crust mixture evenly into the bottom of the prepared pan. Bake for about 8 minutes, or until lightly golden.

4. **Prepare the Lemon Filling**: While the crust is baking, whisk together the eggs, granulated sugar, flour, lemon juice, and lemon zest in a large bowl until smooth.

5. **Assemble the Bars**: Remove the baked crust from the oven. Spread the warm raspberry sauce evenly over the crust. Pour the lemon filling over the raspberry layer; it will naturally swirl together.

6. **Bake**: Return the pan to the oven and bake for 20-25 minutes, or until the filling is set and lightly browned around the edges.

7. **Cool and Serve**: Allow the bars to cool completely in the pan. Use the foil to lift the bars out, then cut into squares. Dust with powdered sugar before serving, if desired.

Cooking and Prep Time

- **Prep Time**: 20 minutes
- **Cook Time**: 30-35 minutes
- **Total Time**: Approximately 1 hour

Servings

- Makes about 16 bars.

Nutrition (per bar, approximate)

- Calories: 180
- Fat: 8g
- Carbohydrates: 26g
- Fiber: 1g
- Protein: 3g
- Sugar: 12g

6.5.14 Chia and Fruit Salad

Ingredients

- 2 cups mixed fresh fruit (e.g., strawberries, blueberries, kiwi, mango, and banana)
- 1 tablespoon chia seeds
- 2 tablespoons honey or maple syrup (optional)
- 1 tablespoon lime juice
- Fresh mint leaves for garnish (optional)

Directions

1. **Prepare the Fruit**: Wash and chop the mixed fruit into bite-sized pieces. If using bananas, slice them just before serving to prevent browning.
2. **Mix Dressing**: In a small bowl, whisk together the honey (or maple syrup) and lime juice. Stir in the chia seeds and let the mixture sit for about 5-10 minutes. This allows the chia seeds to absorb some liquid and expand.
3. **Combine**: In a large bowl, gently toss the chopped fruit with the chia seed dressing until the fruit is evenly coated.
4. **Serve**: Spoon the fruit salad into serving bowls and garnish with fresh mint leaves if desired.
5. **Chill (Optional)**: For a refreshing touch, you can refrigerate the salad for about 30 minutes before serving.

Cooking and Prep Time

- **Prep Time**: 10 minutes
- **Chill Time**: 30 minutes (optional)
- **Total Time**: Approximately 10-40 minutes

Servings

- Makes about 4 servings.

Nutrition (per serving, approximate)

- Calories: 120

- Fat: 2g
- Carbohydrates: 28g
- Fiber: 4g
- Protein: 2g
- Sugar: 10g

6.5.15 Dark Chocolate Almond Clusters

Ingredients

- 1 cup dark chocolate chips
- 1/2 cup lightly salted almonds
- A sprinkle of kosher salt (optional)

Directions

1. **Melt the Chocolate**: In a microwave-safe bowl, melt the dark chocolate chips in 30-second increments, stirring after each interval until fully melted and smooth.
2. **Combine with Almonds**: Add the lightly salted almonds to the melted chocolate and stir until the almonds are evenly coated.
3. **Form Clusters**: Using a tablespoon, scoop out the chocolate-almond mixture and drop it onto a silicone baking mat or parchment-lined baking sheet, forming mounds.
4. **Add Salt**: If desired, sprinkle a little kosher salt on top of each cluster before they set.
5. **Chill**: Refrigerate the clusters for at least 30 minutes to allow them to firm up.
6. **Serve or Store**: Keep the clusters refrigerated until ready to serve. They can also be frozen for later enjoyment.

Cooking and Prep Time

- **Prep Time**: 5 minutes
- **Chill Time**: 30 minutes
- **Total Time**: Approximately 35 minutes

Servings

- Makes about 14 clusters.

Nutrition (per cluster, approximate)

- Calories: 99
- Fat: 7g

- Saturated Fat: 4g
- Carbohydrates: 8g
- Fiber: 1g
- Sugar: 5g
- Protein: 2g
- Sodium: 14mg
- Potassium: 117mg
- Calcium: 52mg
- Iron: 1mg

Chapter 6: Lifestyle and Wellness Tips

7.1 Incorporating Exercise for Optimal Health

Integrating regular exercise into your routine is essential for achieving and maintaining optimal health, especially when following the RH Negative Diet. Exercise complements dietary efforts by enhancing overall well-being, boosting metabolism, and supporting various physiological functions. Here's how to effectively incorporate exercise for optimal health:

1. Set Clear Goals:

- **Define Objectives:** Identify your fitness goals, whether they are weight loss, muscle gain, improved cardiovascular health, or enhanced flexibility. Clear goals help tailor your exercise routine to your needs.
- **Track Progress:** Use fitness trackers or journals to monitor your progress and adjust your routine as needed.

2. Choose a Balanced Exercise Routine:

- **Cardiovascular Exercise:** Incorporate activities like walking, running, cycling, or swimming to improve cardiovascular health, endurance, and calorie burning. Aim for at least 150 minutes of moderate-intensity aerobic activity per week.
- **Strength Training:** Include resistance exercises such as weight lifting, bodyweight exercises, or resistance bands to build muscle strength and support metabolic function. Target all major muscle groups at least twice a week.
- **Flexibility and Mobility:** Add stretching, yoga, or Pilates to enhance flexibility, improve joint health, and prevent injuries. Regular stretching helps maintain muscle elasticity and joint range of motion.

3. Create a Consistent Schedule:

- **Establish Routine:** Set a regular exercise schedule that fits into your daily life. Consistency is key to forming lasting habits and achieving fitness goals.
- **Plan Workouts:** Designate specific times for workouts each week, and plan for different types of exercise to ensure variety and balance.

4. Listen to Your Body:

- **Monitor Intensity:** Pay attention to how your body responds to different exercises. Adjust the intensity, duration, and type of exercise based on your energy levels and any physical limitations.
- **Rest and Recovery:** Incorporate rest days and allow time for recovery between intense workouts to prevent overtraining and reduce the risk of injury.

5. Combine Exercise with Dietary Goals:

- **Nutritional Support:** Fuel your workouts with appropriate nutrition by consuming balanced meals and snacks that align with the RH Negative Diet. Proper hydration, protein intake, and healthy fats support exercise performance and recovery.
- **Timing:** Consider the timing of your workouts relative to meals. Eating a light snack before exercise can provide energy, while consuming a post-workout meal can aid in recovery.

6. Engage in Activities You Enjoy:

- **Find Enjoyable Exercises:** Choose physical activities that you find enjoyable and motivating. Whether it's dancing, hiking, or group fitness classes, enjoying your exercise routine increases the likelihood of sticking with it.
- **Variety:** Incorporate a variety of activities to keep your routine interesting and prevent boredom. Mixing different types of exercise also ensures a well-rounded fitness regimen.

7. Incorporate Functional Movements:

- **Daily Activities:** Include exercises that mimic everyday movements to improve functional fitness. Activities like squats, lunges, and balance exercises enhance your ability to perform daily tasks with ease.

8. Seek Professional Guidance:

- **Personal Trainer:** If you're new to exercise or have specific fitness goals, consider working with a personal trainer for customized guidance and support.
- **Exercise Programs:** Explore reputable fitness programs or apps that offer structured workout plans and instructional content.

By incorporating these strategies into your routine, you can optimize your health and complement the benefits of the RH Negative Diet. Regular exercise not only supports physical health but also contributes to mental well-being, energy levels, and overall quality of life.

7.2 Stress Management Techniques

Effective stress management is crucial for maintaining overall health and enhancing the benefits of the RH Negative Diet. Chronic stress can negatively impact metabolism, digestion, and immune function. Incorporating stress management techniques into your daily routine can help reduce stress levels and improve well-being. Here are some proven strategies:

1. Mindfulness and Meditation:

- **Mindfulness Practice:** Engage in mindfulness techniques to stay present and focused. Simple practices, such as mindful breathing or paying attention to sensory experiences, can help manage stress and increase relaxation.
- **Meditation:** Incorporate meditation sessions into your routine to calm the mind and reduce stress. Techniques such as guided meditation, loving-kindness meditation, or body scan meditation can be effective.

2. Physical Activity:

- **Exercise Regularly:** Physical activity helps release endorphins, which are natural mood lifters. Incorporate activities like walking, jogging, or yoga to alleviate stress and boost overall mental health.
- **Active Relaxation:** Engage in activities that combine exercise with relaxation, such as tai chi or gentle yoga, to reduce stress and improve flexibility.

3. Healthy Eating Habits:

- **Balanced Diet:** Follow a balanced diet that supports overall health and well-being. Consuming nutrient-dense foods can help stabilize blood sugar levels and improve mood.
- **Hydration:** Stay well-hydrated, as dehydration can exacerbate stress and affect cognitive function. Aim to drink plenty of water throughout the day.

4. Adequate Sleep:

- **Establish a Routine:** Create a consistent sleep schedule by going to bed and waking up at the same times each day. Quality sleep is essential for stress management and overall health.
- **Create a Restful Environment:** Ensure your sleep environment is conducive to rest by maintaining a cool, dark, and quiet room. Avoid screens and stimulating activities before bedtime.

5. Relaxation Techniques:

- **Deep Breathing:** Practice deep breathing exercises to calm the nervous system and reduce stress. Techniques such as diaphragmatic breathing or the 4-7-8 method can be effective.
- **Progressive Muscle Relaxation:** Use progressive muscle relaxation to release physical tension. This involves tensing and then relaxing different muscle groups systematically.

6. Social Support:

- **Connect with Others:** Build and maintain strong social connections with family, friends, or support groups. Sharing experiences and seeking support can help alleviate stress and provide emotional relief.
- **Communicate:** Openly communicate your feelings and concerns with trusted individuals to gain perspective and reduce stress.

7. Time Management:

- **Prioritize Tasks:** Organize and prioritize tasks to manage your time effectively. Break larger tasks into smaller, manageable steps and set realistic deadlines.
- **Set Boundaries:** Establish boundaries to avoid overcommitting and ensure you have time for relaxation and self-care.

8. Engage in Hobbies and Interests:

- **Pursue Enjoyable Activities:** Engage in hobbies and activities that bring joy and fulfillment. Activities such as reading, painting, or gardening can provide a positive outlet for stress.

9. Professional Help:

- **Seek Counseling:** If stress becomes overwhelming or persistent, consider seeking professional help from a therapist or counselor. They can provide coping strategies and support for managing stress effectively.
- **Stress Management Programs:** Explore stress management programs or workshops that offer structured techniques and support.

Incorporating these stress management techniques into your routine can help you maintain balance and resilience, supporting the effectiveness of the RH Negative Diet and contributing to overall health and well-being.

7.3 Sleep and Its Impact on Your Diet

Sleep plays a crucial role in overall health and directly impacts dietary habits and metabolic processes. Quality sleep is essential for maintaining a balanced diet and achieving optimal health, especially when following the RH Negative Diet. Here's how sleep influences your diet and strategies to improve sleep for better health outcomes:

1. Effects of Sleep on Metabolism:

- **Regulation of Hunger Hormones:** Adequate sleep helps regulate hormones that control hunger, such as ghrelin (which stimulates appetite) and leptin (which signals fullness). Poor sleep can lead to increased hunger and cravings, often for high-calorie, sugary foods.
- **Impact on Insulin Sensitivity:** Lack of sleep can impair insulin sensitivity, leading to difficulties in glucose metabolism and an increased risk of weight gain and metabolic disorders.

2. Sleep and Food Choices:

- **Increased Cravings:** Sleep deprivation is associated with heightened cravings for unhealthy foods, including those high in sugar and fat. This can result in poor dietary choices and overeating.
- **Disrupted Satiety:** Poor sleep can disrupt the body's ability to recognize and respond to hunger and fullness cues, potentially leading to overeating or frequent snacking.

3. Quality of Sleep and Digestive Health:

- **Digestive Function:** Good sleep supports healthy digestive function by allowing the body to properly process and absorb nutrients. Inadequate sleep can lead to digestive issues such as bloating or acid reflux.

- **Meal Timing:** Eating large meals close to bedtime can interfere with sleep quality. It's beneficial to allow a few hours between your last meal and bedtime to promote restful sleep.

4. Strategies for Improving Sleep:

- **Establish a Routine:** Create a consistent sleep schedule by going to bed and waking up at the same times each day. Consistency helps regulate your internal clock and improves sleep quality.
- **Create a Relaxing Environment:** Ensure your sleep environment is conducive to rest. Maintain a cool, dark, and quiet room, and use comfortable bedding to promote better sleep.
- **Limit Stimulants:** Avoid consuming caffeine, nicotine, and large amounts of alcohol, particularly in the hours leading up to bedtime. These substances can disrupt sleep patterns and reduce sleep quality.

5. Enhancing Sleep Hygiene:

- **Pre-Sleep Routine:** Develop a calming pre-sleep routine that includes activities such as reading, gentle stretching, or practicing relaxation techniques. Avoid screens and stimulating activities before bed.
- **Manage Stress:** Incorporate stress management techniques, such as mindfulness or deep breathing, to reduce anxiety and promote relaxation before sleep.

6. Impact on Dietary Habits:

- **Mindful Eating:** Pay attention to your body's hunger and fullness signals to avoid emotional or stress-related eating. Quality sleep supports better decision-making and portion control.
- **Balanced Meals:** Maintain a balanced diet with regular meals and snacks to stabilize blood sugar levels and prevent excessive hunger or cravings.

7. Addressing Sleep Disorders:

- **Seek Professional Help:** If you experience chronic sleep issues, such as insomnia or sleep apnea, consult a healthcare professional. They can provide appropriate diagnosis and treatment options to improve sleep quality.

By recognizing and addressing the relationship between sleep and diet, you can enhance both your sleep quality and dietary adherence. Prioritizing good sleep practices supports metabolic health, optimal nutrient utilization, and overall well-being, making it an integral part of a successful RH Negative Diet.

Chapter 7: Troubleshooting and FAQs

8.1 Common Challenges and Solutions

Following the RH Negative Diet may present several challenges, but understanding and addressing these issues can help you stay on track and achieve your health goals. Here are some common challenges and practical solutions:

1. Challenge: Adherence to Dietary Restrictions

- **Solution:** Plan meals in advance and keep a well-stocked pantry with approved foods. Use meal prepping and batch cooking to make sticking to the diet easier.

2. Challenge: Limited Food Variety

- **Solution:** Explore new recipes and try different foods within the allowed categories. Incorporate diverse cooking methods and seasonings to add variety.

3. Challenge: Eating Out or Social Situations

- **Solution:** Review restaurant menus ahead of time and choose dishes that fit your dietary needs. Communicate your requirements to hosts or servers when attending social events.

4. Challenge: Nutrient Deficiencies

- **Solution:** Ensure a well-balanced intake of nutrients by including a variety of allowed foods. Consider consulting with a dietitian for personalized advice and supplementation if needed.

5. Challenge: Overcoming Cravings for Restricted Foods

- **Solution:** Find healthy alternatives and satisfying substitutes that align with the RH Negative Diet. Focus on the benefits of the diet and how it supports your overall health goals.

By proactively addressing these challenges, you can maintain adherence to the RH Negative Diet and achieve long-term success.

8.2 How to Adjust the Diet for Specific Health Conditions

Adjusting the RH Negative Diet to address specific health conditions can help manage symptoms and improve overall health. Tailoring the diet to individual needs ensures that it supports rather than hinders your well-being. Here's how to modify the diet for various health conditions:

1. Diabetes:

- **Focus on Low Glycemic Foods:** Choose foods with a low glycemic index to help stabilize blood sugar levels. Opt for whole grains, legumes, and non-starchy vegetables.
- **Monitor Carbohydrate Intake:** Pay attention to portion sizes and balance carbohydrates with proteins and fats to avoid blood sugar spikes.
- **Incorporate Fiber:** Include high-fiber foods like leafy greens, nuts, and seeds to support blood sugar control and improve digestion.

2. Heart Disease:

- **Emphasize Healthy Fats:** Include sources of omega-3 fatty acids, such as fatty fish (salmon, mackerel) and flaxseeds, to support heart health.
- **Limit Saturated Fats and Cholesterol:** Reduce intake of high-fat meats and dairy products. Opt for lean proteins and plant-based alternatives.
- **Increase Antioxidant-Rich Foods:** Incorporate fruits and vegetables rich in antioxidants, like berries and leafy greens, to help reduce inflammation and support cardiovascular health.

3. Digestive Disorders (e.g., IBS, Crohn's Disease):

- **Identify Trigger Foods:** Keep a food diary to identify and avoid specific foods that trigger symptoms. Common triggers include high-FODMAP foods and certain dairy products.

- **Focus on Digestive Health:** Include easily digestible foods and fiber sources that promote gut health, such as cooked vegetables and probiotic-rich foods (e.g., yogurt, fermented foods).

4. Autoimmune Conditions:

- **Follow an Anti-Inflammatory Diet:** Incorporate anti-inflammatory foods like turmeric, ginger, and omega-3-rich fish. Avoid foods that can trigger inflammation, such as processed foods and high-sugar items.
- **Consider Elimination Protocols:** For conditions like rheumatoid arthritis or lupus, consider elimination diets to identify and remove specific allergens or irritants from your diet.

5. Weight Management:

- **Monitor Portion Sizes:** Be mindful of portion sizes to help manage calorie intake and support weight loss or maintenance.
- **Balance Macronutrients:** Ensure meals are balanced with proteins, healthy fats, and complex carbohydrates to promote satiety and reduce overeating.

6. Thyroid Disorders (e.g., Hypothyroidism, Hyperthyroidism):

- **Include Iodine-Rich Foods:** For hypothyroidism, include iodine-rich foods such as seaweed and iodized salt. However, avoid excess iodine as it can affect thyroid function.
- **Monitor Goitrogenic Foods:** If you have thyroid issues, be cautious with goitrogens (e.g., raw cruciferous vegetables) that can affect thyroid function. Cooking these foods can reduce their goitrogenic effects.

7. Bone Health:

- **Increase Calcium and Vitamin D:** Include calcium-rich foods like leafy greens and fortified plant-based milks, and ensure adequate vitamin D intake through sunlight exposure or supplements.

- **Support Bone Density:** Incorporate foods rich in magnesium and vitamin K, which are important for bone health.

8. Allergies and Sensitivities:

- **Avoid Allergens:** Clearly identify and avoid foods that cause allergic reactions or sensitivities. Replace with suitable alternatives that meet dietary needs.
- **Read Labels:** Carefully read food labels to avoid hidden allergens and irritants in processed foods.

Adjusting the RH Negative Diet to accommodate specific health conditions requires careful planning and personalized modifications. Consulting with a healthcare provider or dietitian can provide additional guidance tailored to your individual health needs and goals.

8.3 Final Though

Embarking on the RH Negative Diet is a journey towards better health and well-being, tailored to the unique needs of individuals with RH negative blood types. As you navigate this diet, it's essential to remember that flexibility and personalization are key to achieving long-term success.

1. Embrace Personalization:

- **Adapt and Modify:** The RH Negative Diet provides a framework, but personal adjustments may be necessary to fit individual health conditions, preferences, and lifestyle. Tailoring the diet to your specific needs can enhance its effectiveness and sustainability.
- **Listen to Your Body:** Pay attention to how your body responds to different foods and meal patterns. Adjust your diet based on your observations and experiences.

2. Prioritize Balanced Nutrition:

- **Focus on Nutrient-Dense Foods:** Aim for a balanced intake of proteins, healthy fats, carbohydrates, vitamins, and minerals. A diverse and nutrient-rich diet supports overall health and helps prevent deficiencies.
- **Maintain Variety:** Incorporate a wide range of foods to ensure you receive comprehensive nutrition and avoid dietary monotony.

3. Incorporate Holistic Practices:

- **Combine with Healthy Lifestyle Choices:** Complement the RH Negative Diet with regular exercise, stress management, and adequate sleep. These holistic practices enhance the benefits of the diet and contribute to overall well-being.

- **Seek Professional Guidance:** For personalized advice and support, consider consulting with a healthcare provider or dietitian. They can help address specific health concerns and provide tailored recommendations.

4. Stay Informed and Adaptable:

- **Keep Learning:** Stay informed about the latest research and developments related to blood type diets and nutrition. Being knowledgeable allows you to make informed decisions and adjustments.
- **Be Flexible:** Understand that maintaining a healthy diet is a dynamic process. Be prepared to make changes and adapt as your health needs and circumstances evolve.

5. Celebrate Progress:

- **Acknowledge Achievements:** Recognize and celebrate your progress and achievements along the way. Small victories and improvements in health and well-being are important milestones.
- **Stay Motivated:** Keep your health goals in mind and stay motivated by focusing on the positive impacts of the RH Negative Diet on your overall quality of life.

By embracing these final thoughts, you can successfully integrate the RH Negative Diet into your lifestyle and achieve your health and wellness goals. Remember that this journey is about finding what works best for you and making informed choices that support your long-term health and happiness.